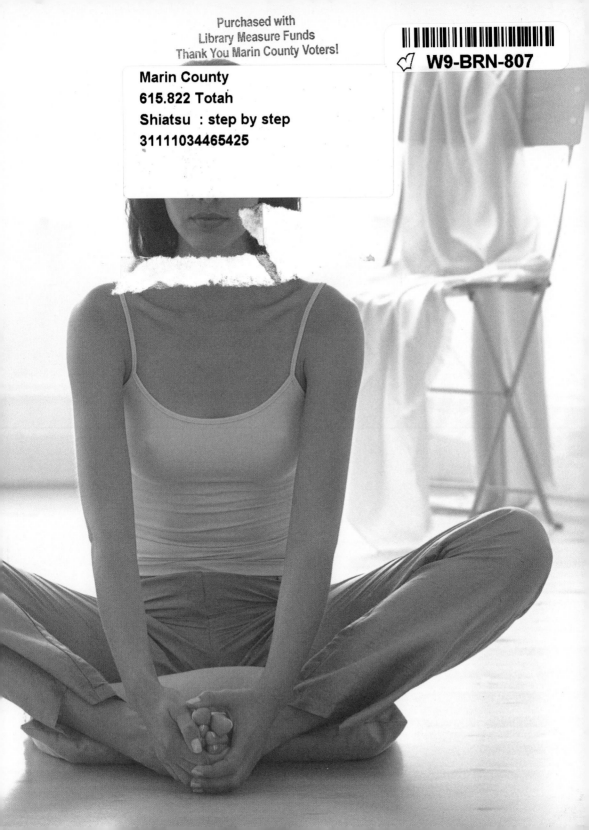

SHIATSU
STEP BY STEP

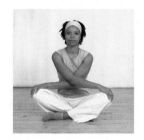

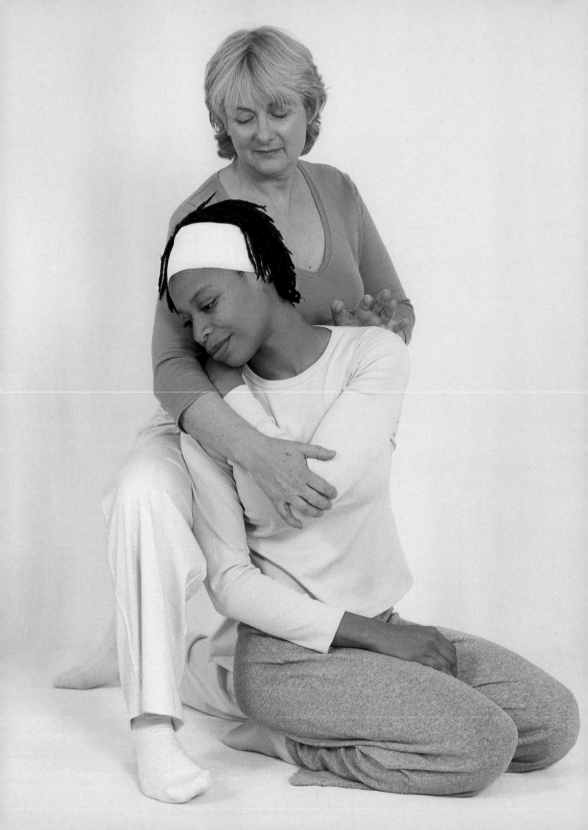

SHIATSU
STEP BY STEP

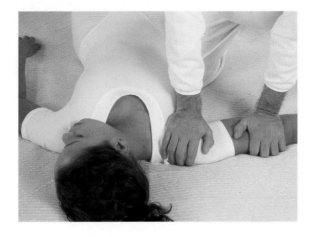

How to unlock and rebalance the body's vital
energy, shown in more than 300 photographs

HILARY TOTAH

WITH FOREWORD BY SAUL GOODMAN

LORENZ BOOKS

Dedication
To Edward Totah, without whom I would never have started on
this road and who gave me so much.

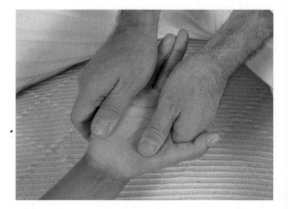

This edition is published by Lorenz Books,
an imprint of Anness Publishing Ltd,
Blaby Road, Wigston, Leicestershire LE18 4SE;
info@anness.com

www.lorenzbooks.com; www.annesspublishing.com

If you like the images in this book and would like to investigate
using them for publishing, promotions or advertising, please visit
our website www.practicalpictures.com for more information.

© Anness Publishing Ltd 2013

A CIP catalogue record for this book is available from the
British Library.

Publisher: Joanna Lorenz
Project Editors: Jennifer Mussett and Emma Clegg
Designer: Jane Coney
Jacket Design: Nigel Partridge
Photography: Clare Park
Illustrator: Sam Elmhurst

The author and publishers have made every effort to ensure that all
instructions contained within this book are accurate and safe, and
cannot accept liability for any resulting injury, damage or loss to
persons or property, however it may arise. If you do have any special
needs or problems, consult a doctor or other qualified professional.
This book cannot replace medical consultation and should be used
in conjunction with professional advice. You should not attempt
Shiatsu without training from a properly qualified practitioner.

Contents

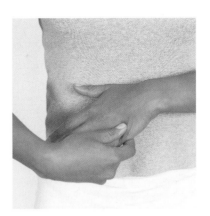

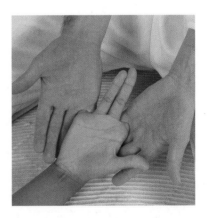

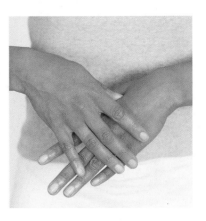

Foreword by Saul Goodman

Since its introduction to the Western world in the 1950s, Shiatsu has become widely recognized as one of the most effective body, mind and spirit therapies. The name comes from *shi*, meaning finger, and *atsu*, meaning pressure. Shiatsu has its roots in the traditions of China and Japan and it incorporates the principles of traditional Eastern medicine and the deeper concepts of chi – the life force.

Shiatsu is recognized by many doctors throughout the world as an effective treatment for various ailments. It is widely used in pre- and post-surgical care, and for pain and physical relief in serious illness and trauma. Trials are also in progress to ascertain the benefits to long-term health conditions, such as arthritis, migraine and digestive problems.

Many psychologists see Shiatsu as an indispensable component in the treatment of emotional and behavioural problems. Shiatsu's growing therapeutic reputation has attracted many people with conditions varying from physical ailments to emotional and psychological difficulties.

Shiatsu has demonstrated more than just a strong therapeutic quality. It has repeatedly shown an enigmatic ability to bring people of all backgrounds together over positive common interests such as growth, well-being and harmony. In the last 25 years a global network of practitioners has organically formed, and is now reaching out throughout the whole world. This network has become a motivating voice in the pursuit of healthy and balanced living

Below Shiatsu practitioners throughout the world follow the same course of assessment, diagnosis and treatment.

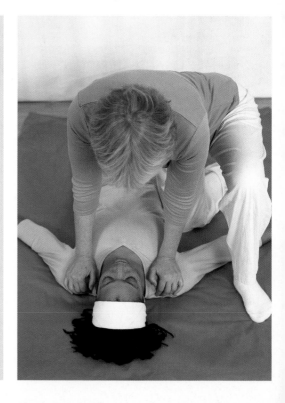

Saul's biography
The Shiatsu specialist Saul Goodman is the founder and director of the International School of Shiatsu, a group of independent Shiatsu schools located in the United States, Switzerland, Italy, Austria, Belgium, Germany, Spain, Portugal and Croatia. He has been practising and teaching Shiatsu and bodywork since 1977.

Saul's unique style of teaching blends the experience of energetics with Western physiology and science. He has inspired many people throughout the world to discover the benefits of practising Shiastu. His first book, *The Book of Shiatsu*, was published in 1986. His other books include

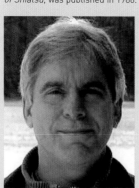

Shiatsu/Shin Tai exploring a form of bodywork known as Shin Tai, *Life Force Recovery*, and *Light Body Activation*. He is based near Philadelphia in the USA.

Left Saul Goodman is an international Shiatsu teacher widely recognized for his inspirational teaching methods.

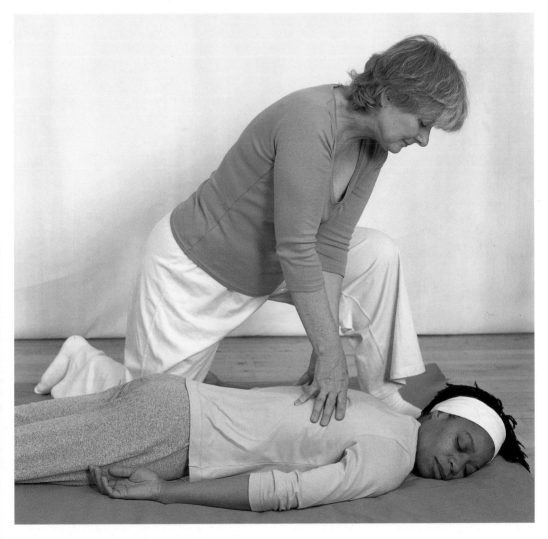

Above Shiatsu relaxes the body and mind and attempts to unlock and bring into balance the energies of the body, encouraging harmony, good health and well-being.

for individuals, families and organizations. Shiatsu has now become a cornerstone of expanding awareness, influencing positive cultural change for the future.

In recent years, due to licensing and professional scrutiny, a large number of Shiatsu practitioners have moved in a more technical and conceptual direction. This is an important factor in creating an interface with the medical and public healthcare communities.

At the same time, no matter how much is explained and analysed intellectually about Shiatsu, the real power of this work lies in its original simplicity. Essentially, this is the

hand, as an extension of the heart, touching another person with care and empathy. This interaction has an almost magical ability to restore a sense of well-being, no matter what the explanation about how and why it works.

This book, by one of my oldest Shiatsu friends, Hilary Totah, gives a fresh and clear perspective about the foundation and practice of Shiatsu. It maintains a strong connection to Shiatsu's essential simplicity. The book is a great beginning for aspiring students, and a good reference for practitioners and teachers. It is written by a person who has a great deal of life experience as a mother, Shiatsu practitioner, school director and author.

Hilary has persistently strived to give her skills generously to the world around her and through this book she makes another valuable contribution.

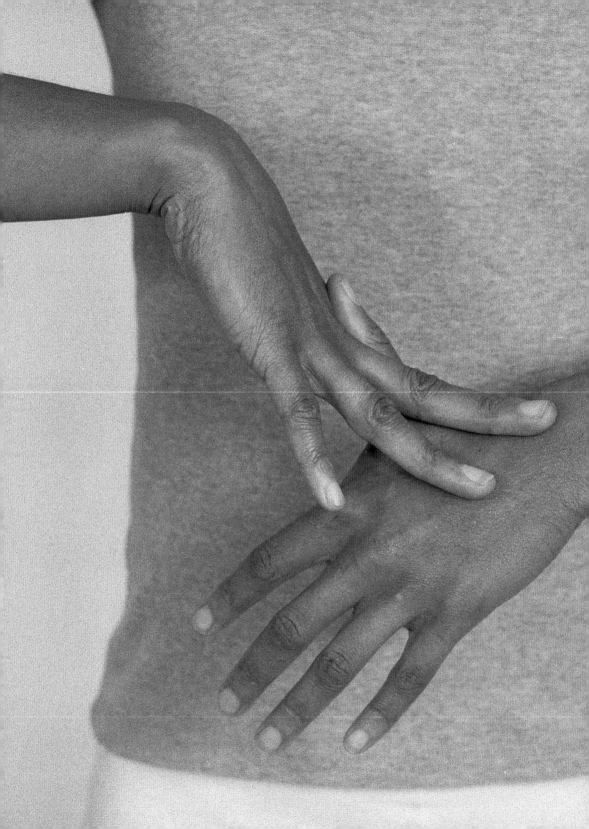

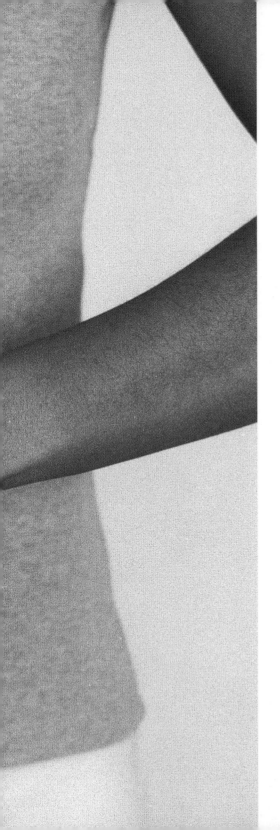

The Beginnings

Fundamental to Eastern medicine is the principle of vital energy flowing through the body, known as chi. The smooth and balanced flow of this energy is thought to be essential to good health and longevity.

Shiatsu works on this vital energy and through the simple application of touch can restore a harmonious balance to the chi flow. Blockages or energy imbalances can be caused by physical, mental or emotional problems and Shiatsu aims to uncover how these factors affect the chi and the treatment needed in order to re-establish balance. Shiatsu will strengthen the body's own innate healing power and will improve health, vitality and well-being.

Understanding the origins and some of the principles of Traditional Chinese Medicine forms the first step to learning and appreciating the art of Shiatsu and discovering how it can help you in everyday life.

What is Shiatsu?

Shiatsu is a traditional healing art from Japan, using touch and pressure to release and rebalance the energy of the body. It is both a form of physical therapy and a means to greater integration of body, mind and spirit. Based on traditional Eastern principles, Shiatsu works on the energetic system of the body, through energy pathways, known as meridians, to bring balance and harmony on a mental, emotional and spiritual level.

The power of Shiatsu is in the use of touch – maybe the oldest form of healing there is. Touch is a comfort, seen every day when a child falls and hurts itself and is soothed by the mother "rubbing it better", or when a hug is shared between friends in times of emotional stress. Touch is as essential a nutrient as food and water for both physical and mental health, nourishing a feeling of trust and of security and belonging. A baby needs to be held to develop a sense of safety and of being loved, and in the same way in adulthood touch can be soothing, healing, and provide an effective method of letting go.

The Japanese word Shiatsu literally means "finger pressure" and a Shiatsu practitioner will use pressure with the thumbs or palms on pressure points and energy

channels of the body to induce deep relaxation. Sometimes the practitioner will use elbows, knees and feet to apply pressure and can give a more dynamic treatment with stretches, massage and mobilization techniques. Receiving Shiatsu brings about a release of tension and leaves the receiver with a sense of being deeply touched and brought back into a state of balance.

The art of Shiatsu depends on the quality of touch of the practitioner, through communication and responsiveness to the client's needs. The practitioner

Below In Japanese, the term Shiatsu means finger pressure. Traditionally, Shiatsu was used as both treatment and as a preventative to encourage good health.

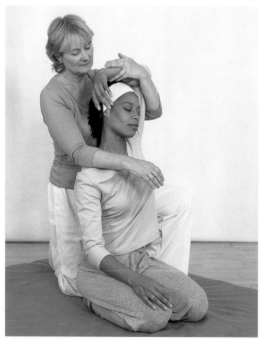
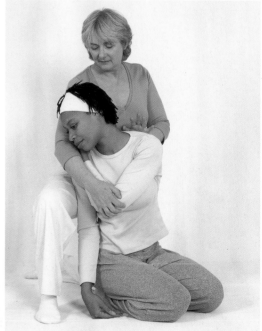

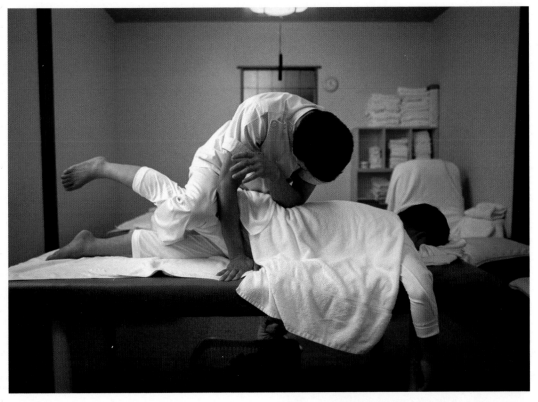

Above The practitioner will use elbows, knees and feet, as well as the fingers and palms, to apply pressure and give a more dynamic treatment of stretches and mobilization techniques.

will use deep, slow holding techniques to work on areas of weakness, and more vigorous techniques, such as rubbing or rocking, on more stiff or tense areas. The practitioner will use their sense of touch as well as observing a person's face, posture, actions and lifestyle to assess how energy may be out of balance and how to bring it back into harmony. Shiatsu combines physical techniques with a finely developed intuition and an understanding of the principles of Eastern medicine, especially the movement and interactions of different energies around the body. These principles supply a framework from which the practitioner can observe and assess the receiver's condition and give an appropriate treatment.

Shiatsu treatment is given with the client lying on a futon mattress on the floor, allowing the practitioner access from all sides and the ability to apply pressure using their body weight with plenty of surrounding space. No massage oils or lotions are required as the practitioner does not move along the body surface, but gives pressure through loosely fitting, comfortable clothing.

Conditions treated

These are some of the more common conditions that a Shiatsu practitioner can treat. Make sure that you advise your practitioner if you would like the treatment to focus on a specific problem or body part.

Traditionally used as both a treatment and a form of preventative medicine, Shiatsu can also be used as part of a healthcare programme or as a form of general relaxation, to rest and recuperate spirit and body.

Headaches	Circulatory problems
Back pain	Anxiety
Neck tension	Depression
Shoulder tension	Stress-related
Stiff muscles	problems
Pulled muscles	Tension headaches
Knee problems	Sleeping disorders
Sports injuries	Tiredness
Digestive problems	Irritable bowel
Menstrual problems	syndrome
Asthma	Childbirth
Insomnia	Pregnancy (not first
Fatigue	trimester)

The History of Shiatsu

Shiatsu is a uniquely Japanese form of therapy, but its roots date back to ancient Chinese philosophical ideas. Four classical approaches to medicine were developed in China. In the south, herbal remedies were readily available. In the east and north, acupuncture and moxibustion were practised, the latter applying heat on chosen points of the meridians. In central China, physical techniques, such as massage and breathing exercises, were used.

In Japan, as travel and trade with China increased during the 10th century, Chinese thought and philosophy, and with them Traditional Chinese Medicine, were becoming more influential. The traditional Chinese form of massage, known as *anmo* (*anma* in Japanese), combined rubbing and pressing on stiff and sore areas and included self-massage

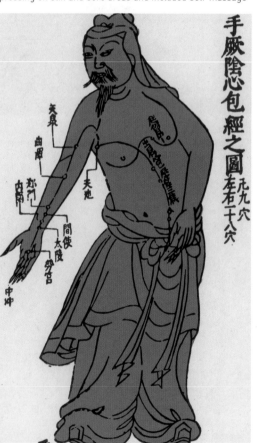

and exercises for detoxification and rejuvenation. By the 17th century Chinese medicine was firmly established in the Japanese culture and the use of anma became widespread. However, over time it lost its medical status and became predominantly a therapy for meditation, relaxation and pleasure.

In the early 20th century, an anma practitioner, Tamai Tempaku, wrote a book called *Shiatsu Ho*, combining anma, *ampuku* (abdominal massage) and *do-in* (self-massage), signalling the birth of the modern-day Shiatsu practised around the world today.

He greatly influenced another practitioner, Tokujiro Namikoshi, who opened the first Shiatsu Institute of Therapy in Hokkaido in 1925. Namikoshi's focus was the legal recognition of Shiatsu in Japan, achieved through acceptance by Western scientific and medical theory. Consequently, all mention of meridians, energy or traditional theory was removed from his work. In its place he required a thorough knowledge of the musculo-skeletal structure and the nervous system, emphasizing neuro-muscular points. He was a popular and charismatic figure in Japan, the author of the book *Do It Yourself – 3 Minute Shiatsu*, which became a best-seller. He appeared on television to promote his technique, using the catchphrase "All you have to do is press". By the 1950s, he had established Shiatsu as an officially recognized and much practised therapy with standard qualifications.

BACK TO BASICS

It was one of Namikoshi's pupils, Shizuto Masunaga, who integrated Shiatsu back into the traditional principles of Eastern medicine, emphasizing the meridians and the Five Element theory (see pages 16–19), which describes the different energy qualities. He was a student of Western psychology and Traditional Chinese Medicine, and was fascinated with the spiritual, psychological and emotional aspects of individuals. He developed his own Shiatsu

Left This Chinese acupuncture chart showing the meridian points dates from AD1031. It indicates the specific medical conditions that can be treated by using each particular point.

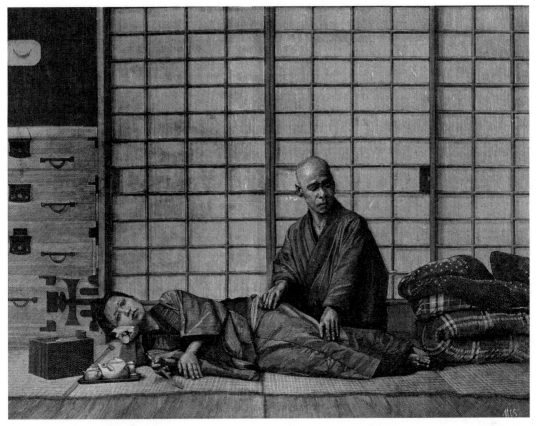

Above This painting dates back to 1896. It depicts a traditional scene with a woman receiving therapeutic massage treatment from a professional Shiatsu practitioner.

bodywork system, later called Zen Shiatsu. Masunaga also developed a form of abdominal diagnosis known as the Hara diagnosis, and extended the traditional acupuncture meridians to include supplementary ones. He established a school in Tokyo called the Iokai School of Shiatsu. His focus on the practitioner's awareness and technique made his system unique and more accessible to the West. He stressed the practitioner's intention, attitude and observation in influencing the treatment, and the importance of using two hands to provide support and connection, creating a more nurturing and less painful experience.

Both Namikoshi and Masunaga came to the West but Masunaga has had the most important influence on Shiatsu today, encompassing more traditional principles and the integration of the psychological and emotional aspects of Eastern medicine. During the late 1970s, one of his students, Wataru Ohashi, brought Masunaga to the United States where he founded Zen Shiatsu, producing a book in English on the subject in 1976. This was the first step towards global popularity. Ohashi describes Namikoshi as the showman of Shiatsu, with his television appearances and popular books, whereas Masunaga was more the intellectual. He attributes Masunaga's popularity in the West to the growing interest in the 1960s and 1970s in all things Eastern and spiritual, whereas Namikoshi was more popular in Japan where the focus was on Western developments and medical advances.

Zen Shiatsu

A sect of Buddhism, Zen focuses on the training of the mind through meditation. The purpose of Zen is to achieve total enlightenment through the discovery of one's basic nature. Its principles and approaches can be applied to numerous human endeavours, including archery, aikido, judo and other martial arts, gardening and architecture, tea ceremony, calligraphy and haiku (Japanese poetry). In the case of Shiatsu, touch is used to balance the body and to reach inner peace. This is achieved through bringing a deep energetic awareness, focused through meridians and points to the part of the body being treated. Emphasis is placed on the inner perception of both giver and receiver.

Chi and the Life Force

The theoretical foundation of Shiatsu uses the concept of the healthy flow and balance of energy, or chi. This idea of energy balance is applied through the body, externally in our environment, and holistically in the way in which we live our lives. Most Shiatsu training involves learning these principles of energy, and understanding how they relate to one another; this enables a much deeper benefit from the Shiatsu experience.

Around the 6th century BC, the Chinese philosopher Lao Tsu wrote the Tao Te Ching, outlining a personal, political and philosophical treatise on a way of living. The Tao, meaning "the way", is an explanation of how the universe came into being. Lao Tsu taught that all straining and striving is counterproductive. One should endeavour to discern and follow the natural forces – to go with the flow of events and not to pit oneself against the natural order of things. This concept underpins all concepts behind Traditional Chinese Medicine. Lao Tsu wrote:

The Tao begat one.
One begat two.
Two begat three.
And three begat the ten thousand things.

CHI ENERGY FORCE

"The Tao begat one" in Lao Tsu's philosophy refers to the chi energy force. Chi, also known as ki or qi, can be translated as "energy" in its widest sense – it manifests in an infinite variety of forms, in air and food, in rock and vibration. It is the source of all movement and change within the universe. Chi never disappears, it just changes form, continually transforming over time. It is essential to life and contained within all living things. Every cell of our body is alive with chi. It is the life force.

Disease, tension and pain are a manifestation of an imbalance or blockage of chi within the body. The work of the Shiatsu practitioner is to bring the chi back to a balanced state through the use of applied pressure on certain areas of the body, based on a correct diagnosis.

The concept of chi is central and is incorporated in many Japanese words: *genki* (good flowing chi) means healthy, while *byoki* (blocked chi) means disease.

YIN AND YANG

Lao Tsu's "One begat two" refers to yin and yang. Over a period of several hundred years, Chinese philosophers differentiated the chi of the Universe into two forces, yin and yang. In Taoist philosophy, the yin and yang symbol represents the two forces that pervade everything in the universe, describing how the universe works, and everything within it.

Chi exercise
In a kneeling position, hold your hands in front of you at elbow height, palms facing each other, about a hand's width apart, as if you were holding a ball. Breathe slowly and attentively. Gently move your hands towards and away from one another several times. Can you feel anything?
Do you experience "something" pushing or pulling between your hands? This feeling or energy can be described as chi.

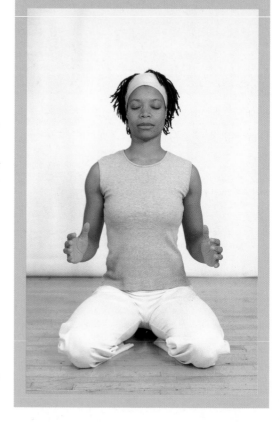

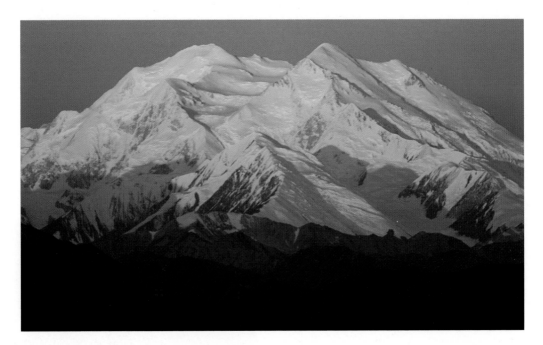

The Chinese used the observation of nature to describe aspects of the world, and the original meanings of the Chinese symbols of yin and yang were the "dark side of the mountain" and the "light side of the mountain". As the sun was seen to move in the sky so the light and dark side of the mountain changed until what was dark became light and light became dark, as all things transform from yin to yang and back again. Things are yin or yang only in relation to other opposite, or balancing, things, such as dark and light, night and day, earth and heaven, front and back, down and up, cold and hot.

Above Mountains were used to describe the qualities of yin and yang; the movement of the sun makes the dark side of the mountain light, as yin becomes yang.

THE YIN/YANG SYMBOL

- The outer circle symbolizes the wholeness and infinity of the cosmos. It contains the yang (light) and the yin (dark).
- Yin and yang are divided by a curved line that represents the movement and constant flow of yin into yang and yang into yin.
- Within the largest portion of each colour there is a dot of the opposing colour. This shows that everything contains the seed of its opposite within it. All things contain both yin and yang energies. There are no absolutes.
- The two colours are in equal proportion, equally balanced. If there is more of one aspect, then there is less of the other, a state of being yin or yang.
- One cannot exist without the other, and all things contain elements of yin and yang.
- All matter, substance and things in the universe are made up of both yin and yang, although at times they may appear to be more influenced by either yin or yang.

The nature of yin and yang

YIN is the quiet, female, intuitive, receiving force, associated with earth. The earth is the source of life, it provides us with what we need to survive. Associated with: earth, down, dark, passive, material, female, front, intuition, interior, autumn and winter, stillness, moon and cold.

YANG is the strong, male, creative, giving force, which is associated with heaven. The heaven above us is always in motion and brings about change. Associated with: heaven, up, light, active, vibration, male, back, intellect, exterior, spring and summer, movement, sun and hot.

The Five Elements

The five elements – wood, fire, earth, metal and water – are the basic building blocks and fundamental components of the universe. Everything in existence contains all five elements but one element will always predominate. The five elements describe the different qualities of chi energy – the five different ways in which it manifests itself in the universe. They represent the cycles in the change from yin to yang and yang to yin.

The origins of the five elements spring from the observation of nature, particularly the cycles of nature. The five elements do not refer to physical elements alone, but to cyclical movements. The name "five elements" can be misleading as it suggests an association with static, immutable properties. Sometimes the theory is referred to as the Five Transformations, which gives a more accurate picture of the fluidity of the cycle.

The theory comprises two aspects. The first is the grouping together of things or phenomena with a similar energy quality, and there are lists of correspondences illustrating this. Listed below are just a few of the major correspondences, which relate to both the natural world, for example the seasons, and the human world, for example tastes and emotions. So you find birth, green and muscles under the wood element and compassion, ideas and humidity under the earth element. The important point is that things that relate to human activity and the activity of nature are woven together when describing the elements.

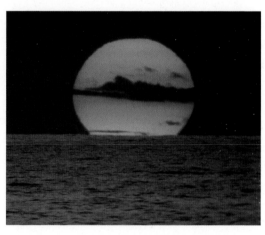

Above The sun provides the fundamental fire energy for the world, affecting the seasonal cycles and the balance of the five elements.

The five elements correspondences

Each of the five elements is imbued with a lengthy list of characteristics, from their colours to the season and body parts and organs. These are used in all practices of Traditional Chinese Medicine to diagnose, harmonize and provide treatment for any imbalances within the system, be it in Shiatsu massage or in feng shui or T'ai Chi. There is an extensive table on pp122–3.

ELEMENT	WOOD	FIRE	EARTH	METAL	WATER
Season	Spring	Summer	Late Summer	Autumn	Winter
Process	Birth	Growth	Transformation	Harvest	Storage
Climate	Windy	Hot	Humidity	Dryness	Cold
Colour	Green	Red	Yellow/Brown	White	Black/Blue
Yin Organ	Liver	Heart	Spleen	Lungs	Kidneys
Yang Organ	Gall Bladder	Small Intestine	Stomach	Large Intestine	Bladder
Tissue	Muscles	Blood Vessels	Flesh	Skin	Bones
Sense	Sight	Speech	Taste	Smell	Hearing
Taste	Sour	Bitter	Sweet	Spicy	Salty
Sound	Shouting	Laughing	Singing	Crying	Groaning
Emotion	Anger	Joy	Compassion	Depression	Fear
Capacity	Planning	Spiritual	Ideas/Opinions	Elimination	Awareness

Right In the natural world, the five elements flow into one another, their interaction moulding together to form the whole.

17

THE BEGINNINGS

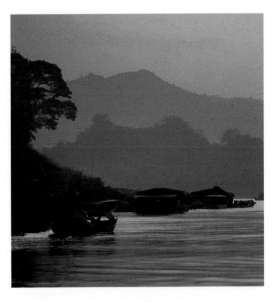

The second aspect of the five elements theory looks at the flow of energy between the elements in a defined sequence. There are two cycles that describe this interaction of the five elements. They are the Creative (Shen) Cycle and the Control (Ko) Cycle.

THE CREATIVE (SHEN) CYCLE
This cycle describes the interaction of the five elements where one element precedes and gives rise to the next one. It illustrates how the energy flows in a circle from yin to yang. Sometimes called the Supporting Cycle, each preceding element, which can be described as the mother, nourishes or supports the following element.

This cycle is clearly manifested in the external world by the seasons. Wood-spring (birth) feeds the fire of summer (maturation) creating the earth-late summer (harvest). Out of earth comes metal-autumn (dying back, letting go) continuing on to water-winter (death, hibernation), which then completes the cycle to regenerate as wood-spring (rebirth). In Traditional Chinese Medicine treatments, a weakness in one part of the body can be treated by boosting the key element for that body part, such as metal for the lung, and also by increasing the element that creates metal, which is earth.

THE CREATIVE CYCLE
One of the two cycles that describes the interaction of the five elements, the Creative Cycle – also called the Shen Cycle – explains how the five elements support and create one another. Each element springs, or is created, from the previous one, as the seasons transform from one to another: spring (wood) turns into summer (fire), which mellows into late summer (earth), then autumn (metal), which finally flows into winter (water).

WOOD produces FIRE
A material that burns easily, without wood there could be no fire. Wood grows upward (growing yang) and generates fire (extreme yang). As spring turns into the bright and dry summer, wood becomes parched, giving way to fire.

WATER produces WOOD
Trees and plants give life and without water the trees would die. Water (yin) flows into wood (becoming more yang). The end of winter feeds the beginning of spring, with the flow of water into new shoots and trees.

METAL produces WATER
When metal is heated it transforms into a liquid, giving rise to water. As metal turns to fluid it becomes more yin. Late autumn it freezes over and becomes the extreme yin of the cold winter months.

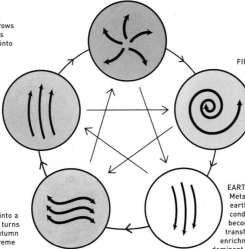

FIRE produces EARTH
As the fire burns out it leaves behind the ashes, which fall and unite with the earth. Fire turns to ashes and settles into earth (yang begins to change to yin). Natural energy flows out of the sun and into the soil as summer dies giving way to the late summer harvest.

EARTH produces METAL
Metal comes from the earth and without earth there would be no metal. Earth condenses (becomes more yin) and becomes metal. As late summer transforms into autumn, with the decay and enrichment of the land, metal becomes dominant.

THE CONTROL (KO) CYCLE

The second cycle that describes the interaction of the five elements is the Control Cycle; this provides a check on the indefinite growth of the Creative Cycle. This is the opposite of the Creative Cycle in that it expresses a relationship where one element exerts control, leading to a suppression that inhibits another element. For example, a metal knife can cut wood and therefore will shape or control it. The Control Cycle is used to prevent one element from draining energy from another. For example, the lung problem that has been treated with Metal (the base element for that part of the body) and Earth (the element that creates Metal) can also be treated by reducing Fire, Metal's controlling element, and allowing Metal to flourish.

The Creative Cycle and the Control Cycle provide a balance that is essential for normal growth and development and also describe the natural balance of chi in the universe. However, when this balance is disturbed the cycles can become distorted. Sometimes the controlled element is too strong or the controlling element too weak and therefore the "natural" order is temporarily reversed. For example, if a fire is fierce and out of control and there is not enough water to suppress it, the water evaporates away.

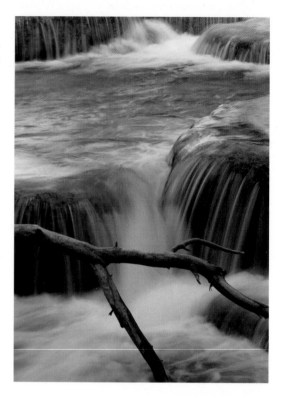

Right Water is the most yin element, representing winter. It flows into wood, in the same way that winter turns gradually into spring.

THE CONTROL CYCLE

This cycle – also called the Ko Cycle – explains how the elements control and reduce the power of one another. If an element becomes too strong, it will cause an imbalance in the whole system. While it will help to create the element next to it, as explained in the Creative Cycle, it will also harm the element after the next, reducing its energy and preventing equilibrium.

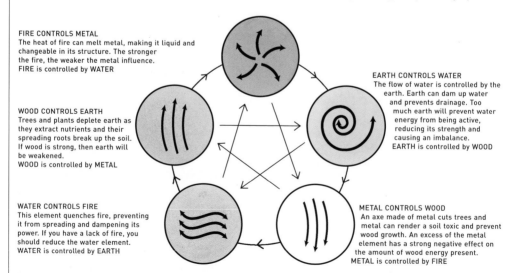

FIRE CONTROLS METAL
The heat of fire can melt metal, making it liquid and changeable in its structure. The stronger the fire, the weaker the metal influence.
FIRE is controlled by WATER

EARTH CONTROLS WATER
The flow of water is controlled by the earth. Earth can dam up water and prevents drainage. Too much earth will prevent water energy from being active, reducing its strength and causing an imbalance.
EARTH is controlled by WOOD

WOOD CONTROLS EARTH
Trees and plants deplete earth as they extract nutrients and their spreading roots break up the soil. If wood is strong, then earth will be weakened.
WOOD is controlled by METAL

METAL CONTROLS WOOD
An axe made of metal cuts trees and metal can render a soil toxic and prevent wood growth. An excess of the metal element has a strong negative effect on the amount of wood energy present.
METAL is controlled by FIRE

WATER CONTROLS FIRE
This element quenches fire, preventing it from spreading and dampening its power. If you have a lack of fire, you should reduce the water element.
WATER is controlled by EARTH

Some common elemental imbalances

IMBALANCE	MEANING	SYMPTOMS
Wood over-controls Earth; Earth becomes weak	Liver (Wood) excess is invading Spleen (Earth) and making it weak	Irritability, diarrhoea, abdominal distension, alternating between diarrhoea and constipation, irritable bowel syndrome, tiredness
Too low Metal cannot support Water	Lung (Metal) is weak and weakens Kidney (Water), grasping Lung chi	Shortness of breath, cough, asthma, lower back ache
Water is weak; Fire out of control	Weakness in Kidney (Water) allows Heart (Fire) to become too hot	Feeling agitated, insomnia, thirsty, high blood pressure, red face
Earth is low; unable to support Metal	Weakness in Lung (Metal) or Spleen (Earth) adversely affects the other	Tiredness, loose stools, weak voice, breathlessness

TREATMENTS USING THE FIVE ELEMENTS

The nature of Traditional Chinese Medicine is holistic – it encompasses the whole life and environment surrounding a person rather than focusing on a specific part of the body. Therefore, when a physical problem occurs, it is viewed as a symptom of a deeper energy imbalance involving the five elements, and is categorized alongside other considerations, such as emotional issues, environmental disharmony or social problems.

The treatment of a disorder is achieved by rebalancing the five elements. As mentioned earlier, this can be done through a variety of therapies, from herbal medicine to the movement therapies of T'ai Chi and Chi Kung. In Shiatsu, meridian pairs relate to each specific element, and by treating these meridians and related points, the flow of the elements can be brought into balance. It is important, when deciding on the meridians to treat, to consider the relationships between the elements according to the Shen and Ko cycles as well as looking at the signs and symptoms in relation to the five elements correspondences.

By looking at the supporting and controlling cycles you can decide which is the element or elements to be treated. For example, if the cause of the condition is weakness in the mother element in the Creative Cycle (as in the example above where Earth is low and unable to support Metal) there will be signs and symptoms in both elements. Earth symptoms are loose stools and tiredness; Metal symptoms are breathlessness and a weak voice. It will be important to treat both mother and child elements to restore balance.

A combination of using the correspondences to see into which element the signs and symptoms fit, and looking at the relationships according to the cycles, can provide a treatment plan to restore health and well-being.

The mother-child analogy

There is a saying in Traditional Chinese Medicine: "If the child screams, treat the mother". The Creative Cycle – also referred to as nurturing – is traditionally seen as the mother-child dynamic. The root cause of the symptoms in the child can be a weakness in the mother where the mother is unable to nourish the child in a wholesome and balanced way. In this case it is important to treat the mother first, as well as treating the child. The Control Cycle is seen as the grandmother-grandchild relationship, where the elders traditionally control the family and keep the young ones in check. If the grandmother is too strict this can lead to a stifling of the child; if she is not strong enough the child may be out of control.

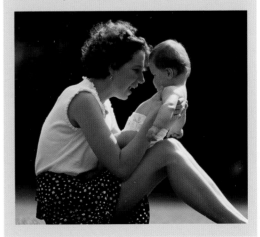

Meridians

Chi energy flows through the body in a similar way to blood, following twelve special invisible pathways or channels that are known as meridians. When chi is flowing freely and in balance through the meridians then a person is healthy. Each of the meridians relates to an organ or organ function. In contrast to Western medicine these are seen as having an emotional as well as a physiological aspect.

The body contains six pairs of vital organs or organ functions corresponding to the twelve meridians, and these perform all the functions of nourishment and sustaining life.

The meridians either carry energy to the organs or carry the energy that the organs produce to other areas of the body. Thus the meridians stretch all over the body, linking apparently unrelated areas such as ears, arms or feet to the vital organs in the centre of the body. In this way, the energy of all parts affects the whole. In meridian theory, chi runs from one meridian to the next in a continuous loop or circuit. The connections between the channels ensure that there is an even circulation of chi, creating a balance of yin and yang. Each meridian pair has a yin meridian and a yang meridian, the yin on the front and the yang on the back.

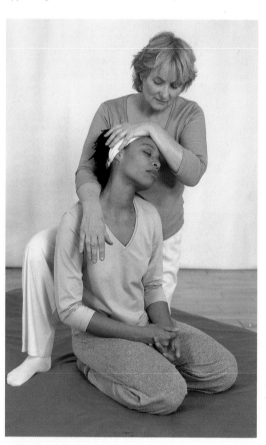

Six pairs of vital organs

Lungs Take in chi during respiration. Symbolizes openness, enthusiasm and positivity. **and Large Intestine** Processes food and eliminates waste. Symbolizes ability to "let go".

Spleen Transforms food into energy. Symbolizes plenty and nourishment. **and Stomach** Receiving and ripening ingested food and fluids. Symbolizes security.

Heart Governs blood. Houses the mind and emotions. Symbolizes joyfulness, calmness and communication. **and Small Intestine** Controls blood and tissue quality. Symbolizes emotional stability, calmness and assimilation.

Heart Protector Protects the Heart, acting as a physical and emotional buffer. Symbolizes harmonious relationships. **and Triple Heater** Maintains homeostasis and symbolizes integration and harmony throughout the body.

Kidney Controls the hormonal system. Symbolizes vitality, courage and the will to move forward in life. **and Bladder** Transforms and excretes urine. Symbolizes qualities of will power and determination.

Liver Stores and distributes blood. Symbolizes creativity, ideas and organization. **and Gall Bladder** Stores the bile. Symbolizes decision-making, flexibility of thought and movement.

Left Shiatsu makes use of stretches, as well as pressure, to release blockages and help the smooth flow of chi through a meridian.

THE FRONT OF THE BODY

The meridians found on the front of the body are the yin meridians (except Stomach, which is yang). They are considered to have a more important role than their yang pair and tend to be more often used in treatment. The front of the body is deep and more to do with maintaining core stability.

Key to the yin meridians

—— Lung

—— Spleen

—— Stomach

—— Heart

—— Heart Protector

—— Kidney

—— Liver

(The remaining meridians are shown on the following pages.)

Pressure points

There are specific points (called *tsubos*) along the meridians where the chi can be more easily accessed, in a similar way to switches on an electrical circuit. These points can be used to help the flow of chi along the meridian, or they can be used to treat specific areas or sets of symptoms. For example, points on the shoulder on the Small Intestine meridian can treat shoulder problems. There are over 700 *tsubos* in the meridian system, each numbered according to the meridian.

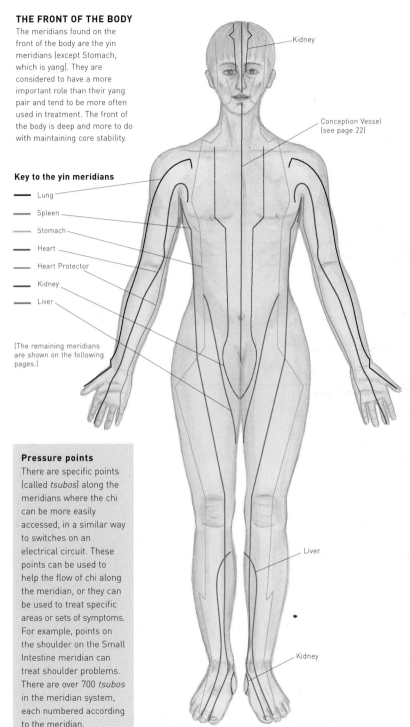

Kidney

Conception Vessel
(see page 22)

Liver

Kidney

Useful pressure points on the front

The pressure points illustrated below and on the next two pages are a selection of important points on the meridians. There are more points illustrated on pages 68–101, provided in the context of the meridians.

Sometimes points can be used to alleviate specific symptoms and the usage given here follows this approach.

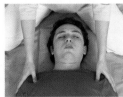

Lung 1
Location: Between the first and second ribs, below the middle of the collarbone.
Usage: Good for coughs, colds and sore throats. Can also help with sinus problems.

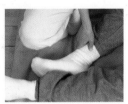

Spleen 6
Location: Four finger-widths above the tip of the inside ankle bone, just behind the shin bone.
Usage: Good for lower abdominal pain, especially period pains. Good for insomnia. Contraindicated during pregnancy.

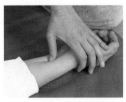

Heart Protector 6
Location: Three finger-widths above the wrist crease on the inside of the lower arm, between the two tendons.
Usage: Good for nausea, especially morning sickness, post-operative nausea and travel sickness.

THE BACK OF THE BODY

The meridians found on the back of the body are yang meridians. The spine is the major structure in the back and represents movement. It is supported by the Bladder meridian and its yu points – major points that relate to each of the body's organs. The yang meridians are more active, transforming, digesting, moving and excreting.

Key to the yang meridians

— Large Intestine

— Small Intestine

— Triple Heater

— Bladder

Triple Heater

Governing Vessel

Large Intestine

Governing Vessel and Conception Vessel

These two channels run through the centre of the body and govern all the yin and yang meridians. The Governing Vessel on the back is called the "Sea of yang", and points on this channel can be used to stimulate the yang energy and to benefit the spine. Points on the Conception Vessel, known as the "Sea of yin", can be used to nourish the yin and help with fertility. They are not used in treatment but they do have important points.

Useful pressure points on the back

These points can be used individually for specific problems or conditions. Apply steady, perpendicular thumb pressure.

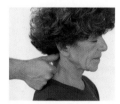

Gall Bladder 20
Location: Below the base of the skull, midway between the mid-line and the prominent bone behind the ear.
Usage: Relieves headaches coming from neck tension and neck pain.

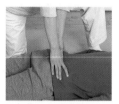

Bladder 23
Location: At the back of the waist between the 2nd and 3rd lumbar vertebrae, one thumb width either side of the mid-line.
Usage: Relieves lower back ache – can be tender, so go in slowly and hold for a while. This point is an important point for the kidneys (known as Kidney Yu point).

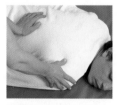

Small Intestine 11
Location: In the centre of the shoulder blade in the depression (you will know when you are on it because it is always a painful point).
Usage: Helps stiff, painful or frozen shoulder, especially at the back of the shoulder.

THE SIDE OF THE BODY

Many of the twelve meridians pass through the side of the body. Gall Bladder, a yang meridian, is the predominant meridian running down the side of the body with important points on the major joints such as shoulder, knee and hip. Joints reflect flexibility and the ability to change direction. Gall Bladder is important in the decision-making process, requiring flexibility and adaptability.

Key to the meridians

—— Large Intestine

—— Small Intestine

—— Triple Heater

—— Kidney

—— Liver

—— Gall Bladder

Movement and the meridians

The meridians in the front of the body, especially the Spleen and Stomach, give stability and support. The meridians at the back, especially Bladder, provide the impetus for movement and spontaneity. A big contributor to back problems is the confusion of these two distinct functions – support and impetus. Shiatsu stresses the importance of strength in the belly or hara to provide support for a healthy spine.

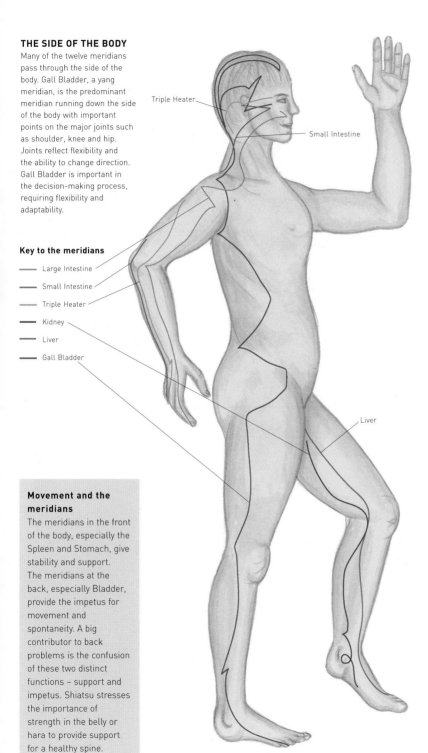

Triple Heater

Small Intestine

Liver

Useful pressure points on the side

These points can be used individually for specific problems or conditions. Apply thumb pressure for one or two minutes.

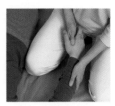

Large Intestine 4
Location: On the back of the hand in the depression where the two bones of the thumb and index finger meet.
Usage: Good for constipation or diarrhoea (known as "the great eliminator"), can relieve toothache and can be used to increase general vitality. Contraindicated during pregnancy.

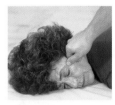

Gall Bladder 1
Location: About one thumb width outwards from the outer corner of the eye in the depression.
Usage: Can relieve headaches behind the eyes and revitalize tired eyes.

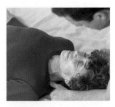

Gall Bladder 21
Location: Midway along the shoulder on the highest point.
Usage: Good for stiff, painful or frozen shoulder, especially on the top of the shoulder. Contraindicated during pregnancy.

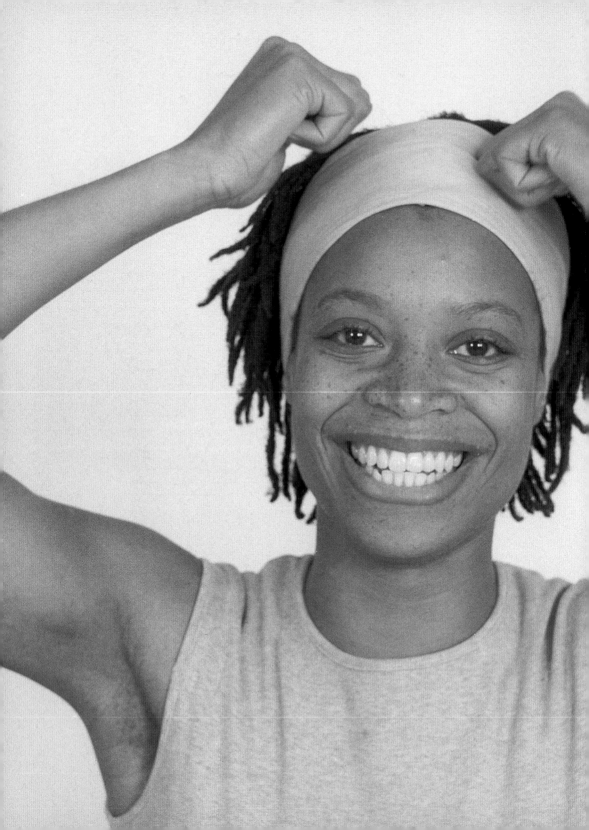

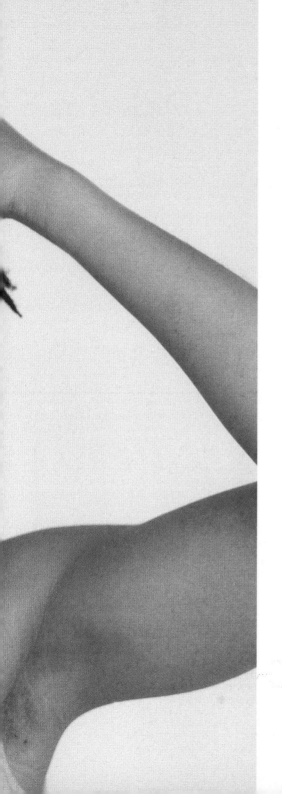

Do-In

Do-in, meaning self-massage, is a set of exercises used to strengthen energy or chi in the meridian systems of the body and in the abdominal area known as the hara. These exercises help to restore balance throughout the whole body, ensuring that the chi is flowing easily and correctly. Do-in includes meridian-stretching exercises, percussion or tapping techniques and breathing meditation.

You can combine the exercises relating to do-in in this chapter – including hara development, energy awareness, self-Shiatsu and makka-ho – to significantly improve your physical and mental well-being. Create your own exercise routine, customized to your own level of fitness and health, to build up strength and awareness. One of the reasons that many people want to learn Shiatsu is to encourage self-healing. This chapter shows you how to develop your body and mind so that your practice of Shiatsu will become easy and enjoyable.

The Practice of Do-In

The following exercises are grouped under different headings and are designed to help in specific areas. Exercises to develop the hara focus on methods of using the breath to centre chi in the hara, as well as exercises to develop hara-centred posture. Energy-sensing exercises use basic techniques to develop an awareness of energy. Self-Shiatsu massage and makka-ho stretches are designed to stimulate the flow of chi throughout the body.

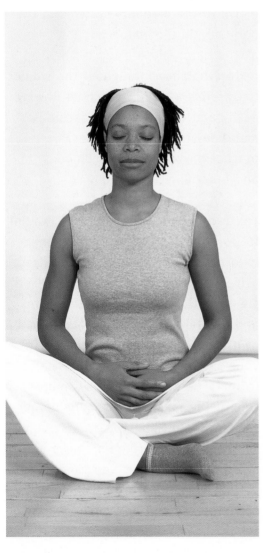

THE HARA

The Japanese word hara literally translated means "belly". The hara usually refers to the abdomen, bordered by the ribs above and the hips and pubic bone below. The centre of the hara is called *tan den*, situated just below the navel, and is also referred to as "one point". The hara is the body's centre of gravity. Energy is stored in the hara, where it is heated before spreading a warm glowing feeling throughout the body.

Hara is an important concept in Japanese culture. To have a good hara is to be healthy. The term for the Japanese tradition of ritual suicide is *hara kiri*, literally meaning "to cut off the hara". The popular sumo wrestlers are incredibly nimble, despite their weight and size, displaying agility and flexibility. The seat of strength is in the big belly, or the hara. In martial arts, the hara is the power centre from which the fighter moves and creates stability and strength.

In Shiatsu the hara is the centre from which we move. The practitioner will allow the body weight to come from the hara. A person with a good hara will stand upright, firm and collected, and will be able to relax their shoulders and be firmly rooted to the ground. With good hara, a person remains balanced both in action and in stillness. There is a sense of security and peace both in body and mind. When based in the hara, we can allow intuition to flow throughout our lives.

In Western cultures people are encouraged to hold the belly in, creating tension and cutting off the free flow of energy in the hara. It helps if you view your belly as the centre of your power. You may find it empowering to think that you have boundless potential energy stored in your hara, and can draw upon it in times of need. It can provide a sense of stability and confidence in everyday life.

Left One of the simplest ways you can develop a sense of hara is by living at floor level. Try moving all the furniture out of the living room, leaving just cushions to sit on. This will increase your flexibility and encourage your centre of gravity to sink. It will also have other benefits, such as helping the digestive system.

Right When you are standing and walking, learn to feel your hara and the energy that it creates. Allow the weight of the belly to drop into the feet and see how stable you become. Feel your hara generating more energy, fuelling your balance and well-being.

ENERGY-SENSING EXERCISES

Shiatsu emphasizes the importance of the vital energy that flows throughout the body using the meridian channels. The energy-sensing exercises in this chapter help practitioners become attuned to their energy flow and initiate the process of rebalancing the body to achieve a freer movement of energy.

SELF-SHIATSU MASSAGE

Self-Shiatsu exercises are a series of massage techniques to restore the flow of chi along the meridians. The exercises in this chapter involve tapping, squeezing, rubbing and pressure to the whole body.

MAKKA-HO STRETCHES

These are a series of six stretches, all of which are similar to yoga postures, stimulating and rebalancing the chi along the twelve primary meridians in the body. The stretches encourage the body to elongate using the breath to let go of tension rather than by forcing the movement. These exercises are frequently used by Shiatsu practitioners to prepare the body for the practice of massage. Using makka-ho stretches will quiet the mind, relax the body, focus attention and improve concentration.

Practising Shiatsu "from the hara"
The art of giving Shiatsu lies within the practitioner's ability to generate chi and move it from the hara. Hara-based work distinguishes Shiatsu from ordinary massage. Here are some benefits of working from the hara.

- The practitioner uses body weight, not muscle power
- The practitioner can relax and physical energy is saved
- There is less risk of injury such as RSI, or "burn out"
- The practitioner uses the whole of their body through the hara to make contact
- The receiver will feel deeply contacted
- The receiver will be more able to relax
- The practitioner will be more in contact with their intuition
- The treatment will flow more smoothly

Before a treatment session, while the receiver is lying on the mat, the practitioner can sit for a few minutes to focus and breathe into the hara to build up chi, let the energy drop to the ground, relax and come up into the body.

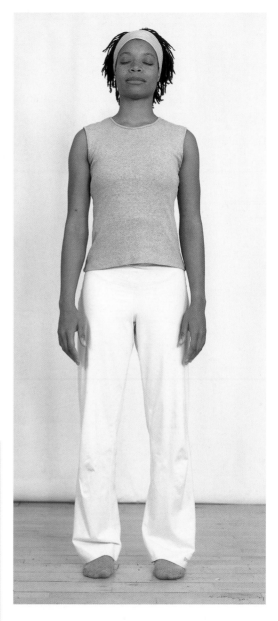

A Shiatsu practitioner will usually recommend specific do-in exercises to individual clients to encourage the flow of energy and to help a particular condition or energy blockage. Practising these Shiatsu exercises will require the ability to move comfortably at floor level. Knees, hips, ankles and wrists should be flexible and shoulders relaxed. Physical strength is not necessary as Shiatsu is given with body weight, but a certain level of stamina and fitness is helpful.

Hara-based Shiatsu

The hara lies deep in the core of your abdomen and acts like a burning flame that brings energy to the rest of your body. Building up the energy in your abdomen by connecting with the hara plays a key role in the warm-up to every Shiatsu session.

Developing the Hara

The exercises that follow are designed to fire up your energy. Close your eyes and focus on your hara, feeling the heat expand through your body. When you feel a tingling, warm sensation in your abdomen, chi is building up and you are ready to begin Shiatsu.

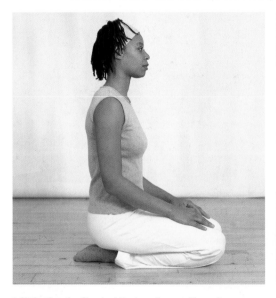

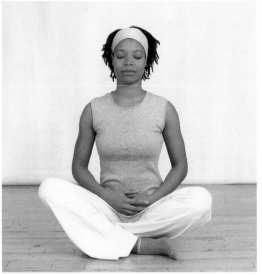

1 Sitting in seiza To adopt the kneeling position, sit on your heels. If this is uncomfortable you can place a cushion between your calves and your thighs. Relax your shoulders and allow the weight to drop to the floor. Gradually increase the time that you sit in seiza until you can sit comfortably for about ten minutes or more.

In Shiatsu, seiza position is used when working on a person's hara, and a wider seiza position is used for other Shiatsu techniques. It is important to be comfortable in this position and feel relaxed while remaining upright.

To focus on your breathing, sit in seiza or cross-legged if you find it more comfortable. (If you are cross-legged you may need to sit on a cushion so that your back is straight.) Close your eyes and relax your shoulders. Observe your breathing calmly and without trying to change it.

2 Breathing into the hara After a few minutes, allow your focus to come to the hara – you may want to place your hands on your belly to help the focus. Gradually encourage your breathing to move down into the abdomen, expanding the belly as you breathe in and contracting it as you breathe out. Imagine your belly is filling with chi as you breathe in and this is dropping to the bottom of the belly. You are getting heavier and your weight is sinking. The belly is filling with chi as you breathe in and you are expelling stale chi as you breathe out. You can imagine the chi as a white light if this helps. Breathe like this for about five to ten minutes, and then gradually allow your focus to come back to the room. Open your eyes and remain sitting for a while. Observe any sensations in your hara – a feeling of warmth, perhaps, or feeling more grounded or heavy.

3 Shifting weight from the hara
Come on to all fours with your hands underneath your shoulders and your knees below the hips. Keep your arms straight. Breathe again into the hara, expanding the belly as you breathe in and contracting as you breathe out. Feel the weight drop evenly between your hands and knees.

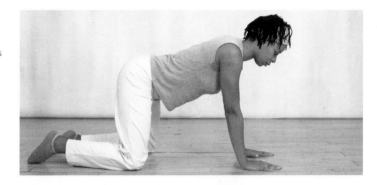

3a Shifting weight from the hara
When you have established your breathing, on the next out breath move your belly forward so that the weight comes more on to the hands. Breathe in and come back to the centre position. Breathe out and this time shift the belly back so that the weight comes more on to the knees. Repeat these two movements.

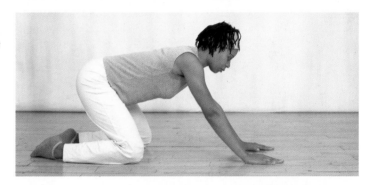

3b Shifting weight from the hara
Begin to make circles with your belly so that the weight shifts first to one hand, then the other, back to the knee on the same side and then the other. Coordinate with your breathing. Repeat a few times and then circle in the other direction.

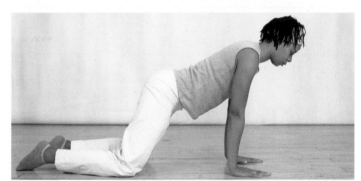

3c Shifting weight from the hara
When you have practised the circling a few times, come back to the central position and breathe again into the hara, feeling the weight drop into your hands. See if you can feel a connection between your hara breathing and the energy in your hands. Come back to seiza, with your hands over the hara.

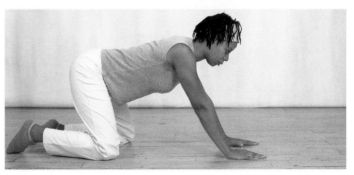

▷

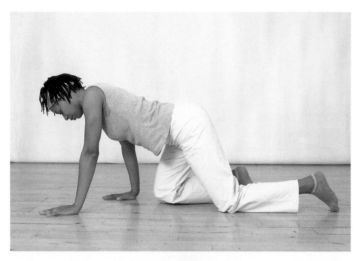

4 Crawling Stay on all fours and crawl around the room as if you were a baby. Move from your hara rather than the hands. Keep your centre of gravity low and concentrate on your hara as you move. Focus on your breath, breathing out as you shift your weight on to your hands. Practise crawling backwards and sideways moving from the hara.

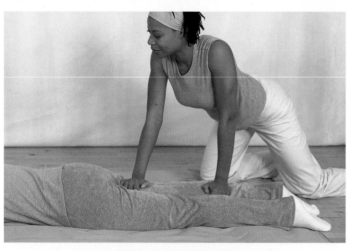

5 Shifting weight with a partner Ask your partner to lie face down on the floor in prone position. Starting from the feet, crawl your palms on to the back of the feet and legs, letting your weight drop into your hands. Work your way up the body on to the back, avoiding direct pressure on the back of the knees and the spine. Make sure that you maintain a relaxed posture, staying open so that the weight always comes from the hara.

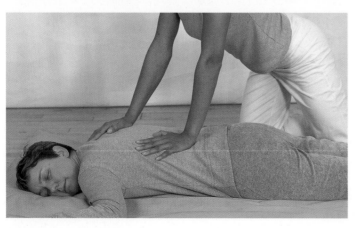

6 Moving your weight Placing your hands in the centre of the back, allow your weight to settle, then shift your weight back and forward by moving your hara in a circular pattern. Slowly crawl your hands down the body, moving your hands down the spine. Don't forget to breathe with your movements, ensuring that the energy is coming from your hara.

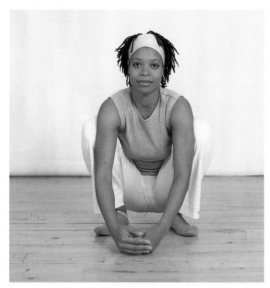

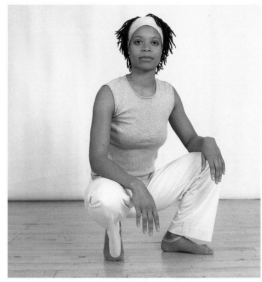

7 Squatting This is a good exercise to increase flexibility in the hips, knees and ankles. While squatting, be aware of your hara and let your weight drop into the feet from the belly. Practise squatting regularly, increasing the time you stay in the position until you are comfortable.

9 Knee-walking (right) This is an aikido exercise that enables the practitioner to move around the client without standing up while remaining in hara. Start in the half squat position. Make sure your stance is not too wide. Let the raised knee drop down and at the same time bring the other foot forward so that you reverse your position. You should find that you move forward. Knee-walk around the room, changing direction. It is better to do this on a carpeted floor or on a padded surface or Shiatsu mat.

8 Half squats This position is a very common one used in many Shiatsu techniques. Squat on the ground with both feet on the floor. Now shift from one side to the other, by lifting one heel then the other. Again be aware of the weight dropping. Practise this exercise regularly.

Crawling
Babies naturally use their hara when crawling. It is thought that a person is naturally aware of the power of the hara from a very young age, and in later life may lose this sense. Next time you see a small baby notice the crawling motion and the use of the belly in the movement. Consider this when you practise on your own.

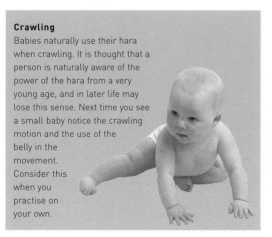

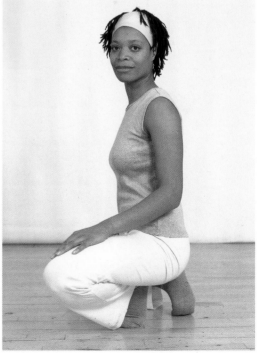

Energy Awareness

Witnessing the flow of energy from the hara to other regions of your body can be both empowering and invigorating. If you have a problem in a specific area, imagine the chi energy flowing in, bringing energy and nourishment.

Tuning in to your Energy

These exercises give you guidance about relaxing and breathing, and about finding the energy in your body. The magnetic energy that you should feel is visualized as an energy ball in your hands; the ball, or rather the chi, is eventually absorbed by the body.

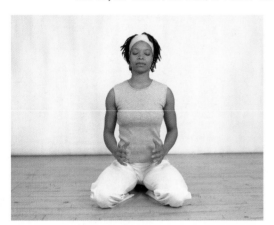

1 Relax and breathe Sitting comfortably in seiza or cross-legged, relax your shoulders and straighten your spine. Bend your elbows and bring your hands in front of your belly, with palms facing. Close your eyes and breathe into your hara, imagining chi filling your hara as you breathe in.

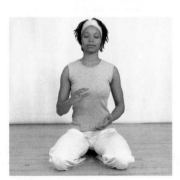

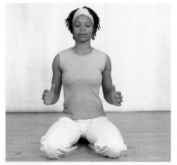

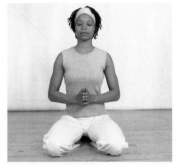

2 Finding the energy Take time to build up energy between your hands. You may be aware of a magnetic sensation on bringing your hands together or pushing them apart. Imagine that this energy is a ball and, keeping your hands on either side, move it around and play with it.

3 Push your hands apart Bring your hands and the energy ball back into the original position and as you breathe out allow the chi to push your hands apart. Gradually, on each out breath, the chi will force your hands to drift apart.

4 Draw back your hands As you take a breath in allow your hands to be drawn back towards each other as if by a magnetic force. Eventually your hands will come back together as the chi disperses between your palms and enters your body.

Do these exercises in the morning, when you want an energy boost, or in the evening to physically and mentally relax and encourage a good night's sleep. The routine should take around forty minutes, although a shortened version can take from five to twenty minutes.

Preparation

Aim to maintain a natural posture and steady breathing and try to keep your mind empty, free of disturbing thoughts. Many people like to focus on their breathing, feeling the air passing in and out of the chest right through to the tip of the nose.

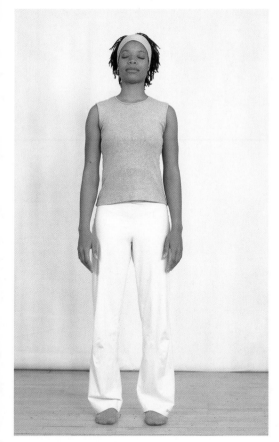

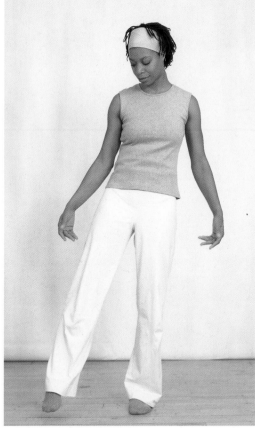

1 Tuning in Stand with your feet shoulder-width apart, knees slightly bent and spine straight. Stand for a few moments, eyes closed, and get in touch with how you feel, being aware of any discomfort in your body and mind.

2 Relax the joints Gently shake out your arms and hands, legs and feet to relax the joints. If you have time, shake out each part of your body separately, starting from your fingers and working down your arms and trunk to your legs.

The Head

Bringing chi to the head is important for waking up the brain and increasing mental clarity. These are good exercises to do first thing in the morning so that you start the day alert. Releasing tension in the neck increases blood flow to the head.

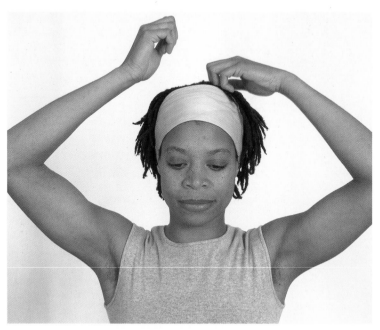

1 Tapping all over the head
Use loose fists to tap all over the head, especially at the base of the skull. This wakes up the brain, stimulating blood and energy flow around the brain and helping you to feel alive and fresh. You can gauge how hard or softly to tap, using your fingertips for a more gentle approach if necessary. Ensure that you tap all over the head, including behind the ears, the top of the head and the base of the skull.

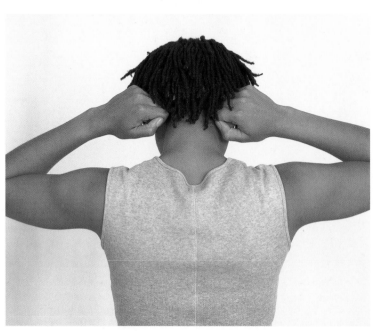

2 Tapping down the back of the neck Open the back of the neck area by lowering your chin down as far as you can, but without over-stretching. Reach your arms right back before you start tapping, opening your chest out and feeling the chi from your hara flowing freely into the head and neck area. Then tap gently all over the area, moving up and down the sides of your neck, avoiding direct pressure on the central vertebrae.

The Arms and Shoulders

Tension in the shoulders and upper arms can prevent the proper circulation of chi around your whole body, and especially into the head area. Make sure that your arms and shoulders are feeling loose by performing the following exercises.

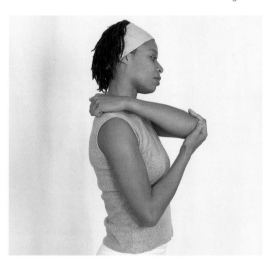

1 Tapping across the shoulders Tap across one shoulder at a time, starting at the base of the neck and moving out to the outside edge, working along the trapezius muscle. Support your elbow with the other hand so that you can reach as far as possible along the back of the shoulder. Spend some time here, tapping away any tension.

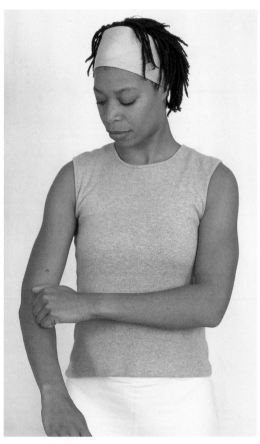

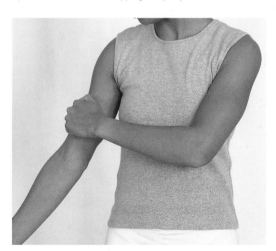

2 Tapping down the inside of the arm Open the arm with palm up and starting from the top tap down towards the hand. This will be stimulating the meridians on the inside of the arm – Lung, Heart Protector and Heart – which all end on the fingers.

3 Tapping up the back of the arm Tap from the wrist up the back of the arm to the shoulder. This will stimulate the meridians on the back of the arm – Large Intestine, Triple Heater and Small Intestine – which all start on the fingers. Repeat on the other side.

Visualization

You can visualize the chi flowing through the body during this exercise. Imagine the energy or chi flowing freely through your arms as you stimulate the meridians. Feel the chi flow down the inside of the arm and up the back of the arm as you tap. Picture the pathway of each arm meridian, changing the line of tapping each time, from outside edge to middle and inside edge, to release any blockages.

The Hands and Wrists

Spend some time working on your hands; these are your Shiatsu tools, so take care
of them. Here are a few exercises to do daily and before giving Shiatsu. They will
bring chi to the hand by activating the meridians and increasing flexibility.

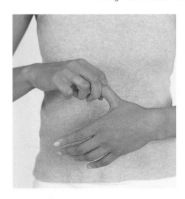 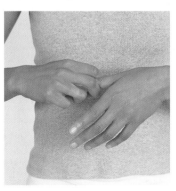 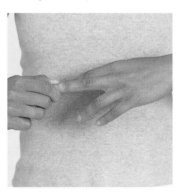

1 Rotate the fingers Rotate and flick the thumb and fingers. Rotate the thumb first one way and then the other. Repeat on the rest of your fingers.

2 Flick the thumb With your thumb and forefinger flick either side of the thumb to the edge of the fingernail. The movement should be performed quickly.

3 Flick the fingers Do the same with each finger, stimulating the beginning and end of each of the meridians that begin or end in the hands and fingers.

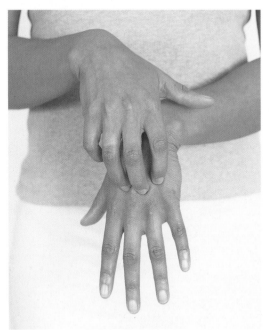 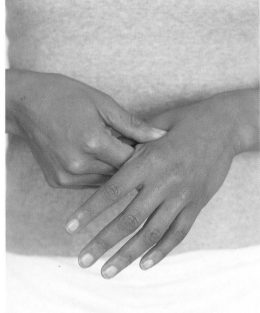

4 Loosen the back of the hand Massage the back of the hand between the metacarpals (the main bones that run through the back of the hands). Work in between the bones of the hands with your thumb and fingers and the tips of your fingers, making space and loosening between the bones.

5 The Great Eliminator Find the point LI 4 (located in the web between the thumb and index finger). This point on the Large Intestine meridian is called the Great Eliminator and is good for increasing vitality and treating headaches, constipation and diarrhoea. Caution: Do not use LI 4 during pregnancy.

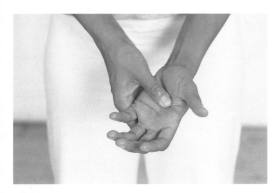

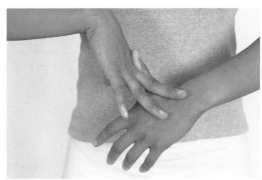

6 Massage the palm Use your thumb to massage HP 8, "the Palace of Anxiety", a good point to calm anxiety and nerves. To find the point, fold your fingers into the palm: the point is where the middle finger touches the palm.

7 Stretch the fingers Using the "V" between two fingers of the other hand as a lever, stretch each finger and the thumb backwards. This will help to increase the flexibility of the hand, making it more adept at performing Shiatsu.

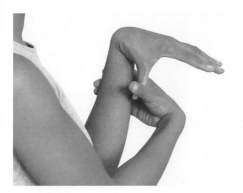

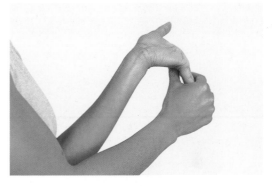

8 Flex and stretch Flex the wrist and stretch the thumb towards the wrist, using the thumb of the other hand. It is important to develop strength and flexibility in the thumbs.

9 Open up the wrist Stretch the wrist open. Bend the wrist back using the fingers of the other hand to exert pressure and open up the wrist. Make sure that you do not overstretch.

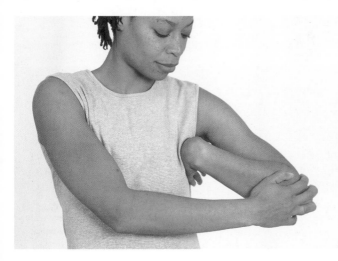

10 Full stretch Stretch the wrist forward. Tuck your hand under the armpit and pull the elbow towards you with the other hand to stretch the wrist forward.

Comparing sides

Do all these techniques on one hand first. Take a moment to compare the hand you have worked to the one you haven't. Notice how it feels. Is it lighter, warmer, more tingling? Find your own words to describe each side. Then repeat all the techniques on the other hand, being aware of the difference between the sides.

The Back and Legs

Loosening the back and legs is a great way to feel energized and increase the flow of chi around your system. Try to reach up your back as far as possible for greatest effect, covering as much area as you can without straining.

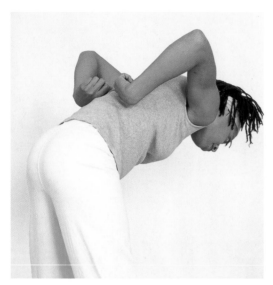

1 Tapping down the back I Bend forward and with loose fists tap down both sides of the spine from the top down to the lower back and then on to the buttocks.

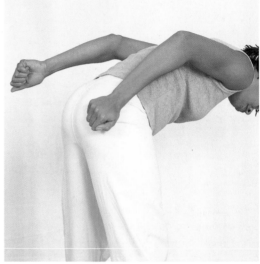

2 Tapping down the back II This process works on the Bladder meridian, the longest meridian, which helps to relax the nervous system and the spine, promoting energy flow.

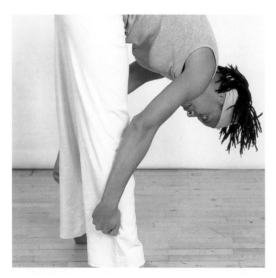

3 Back and sides of legs Tap down the back and outside of the legs and up the inside. Open your feet a bit wider and tap down the back of the legs from the buttocks to the heel, continuing down the Bladder meridian. Bend legs if necessary.

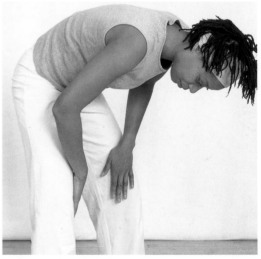

4 Outside and inside of legs With loose fists tap down the side of the legs, then with flat palms tap up the inside of the legs from the ankles to the groin area, paying more attention to the inner thighs – where energy can become sluggish.

The Hara

Releasing tension throughout the hara region allows the chi energy that is generated there to grow larger and become less constricted. Focus on your hara as you apply pressure, feeling the chi energy warming the rest of your body.

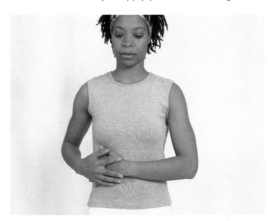

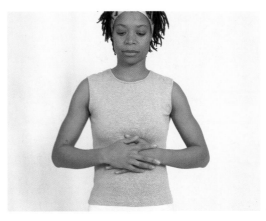

1 Stroke round the hara Finish this Do-in sequence by standing up again with relaxed shoulders and knees. Gently stroke around the hara in a clockwise direction.

2 Stroke the abdomen Use both hands, one placed on top of the other, and stroke around your abdomen clockwise. This follows the direction of the intestines and helps digestion.

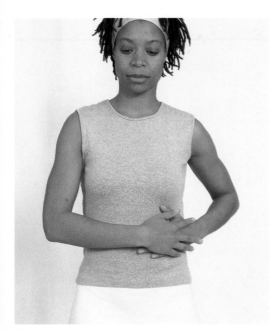

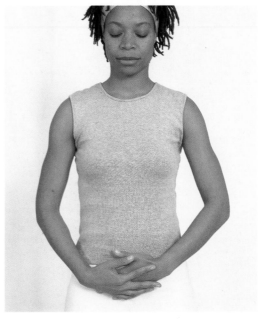

3 Assess changes As you rotate your hands around your hara, take a few moments to get in touch with how you feel now and notice any differences from how you felt at the start of this sequence. Do you feel energized? Did you notice any particularly tense or stiff parts of your body?

4 Stand with both hands on your hara Close your eyes and maintain a relaxed posture, placing one hand over the other and both over the lower part of your hara. Focus your mind on to your hara, imagining it glowing with positive energy and fuelling your whole-body energy system.

Makka-ho Exercises

Each of the makka-ho exercises balances and activates a meridian pair. They can be used as a daily exercise system, and the ease with which you do each stretch also monitors your meridian functioning. A practitioner might recommend a particular stretch to a client based on his or her condition. Start with an in breath and move into the stretch on the out breath. Stay in the position for three or four breaths and on each out breath relax a bit more into the stretch.

The Lungs and Large Intestine

This stretch helps to open up the chest, aiding breathing as well as improving the function of the Lung and Large Intestine meridians. Breathing is a crucial element of good chi circulation. Feel the chi enter with every breath.

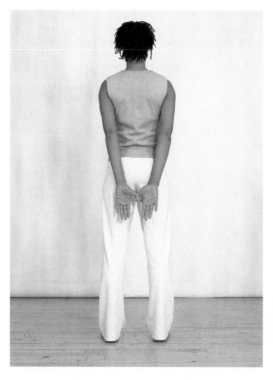
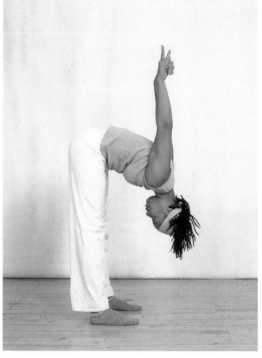

1 Stand and link thumbs Stand with feet hip-width apart. Bring the hands behind your back and link thumbs.

2 Forward and arms up As you breathe out bend forward, bringing your arms up behind you as high as possible and keeping your back and neck straight. Stay for 3–4 breaths, relaxing as you breathe out and feeling your chest open. Come up slowly on the in breath. Repeat with thumbs the other way round.

The Spleen and Stomach

This stretch helps to activate the Stomach meridian on the side of the thighs and helps with digestion. Take care not to overstretch your back and thighs with this exercise. Go down in stages and only go as far as is comfortable.

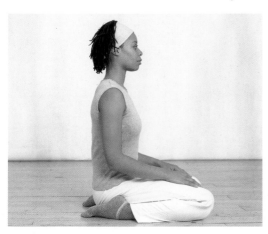

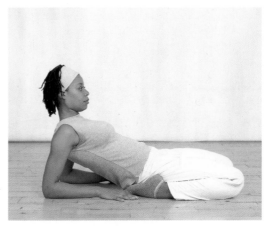

1 Seiza Sit in seiza with your heels on either side of your body, if you can. (If necessary, you can sit on a cushion to ease the hip, knee or ankle joints.) Start with your hands gently resting in your lap, your elbows bent and your shoulders square and upright, looking directly forward.

2 Lean back on your elbows Place your hands behind you, with arms straight, breathe out, lean back and relax. If this is far enough for you, stop here. As you next breathe out, lean back on to your elbows. If this is far enough for you, stop here and breathe into this stretch.

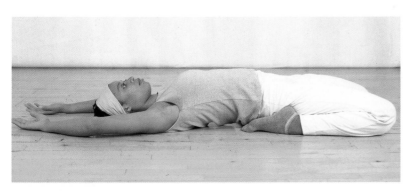

3 Back to floor Breathe out and go all the way back to the floor, raising your hands above your head. Stay here for a few breaths, relaxing into the stretch. If your knees or your lower back come off the floor in this stage come back to the previous position.

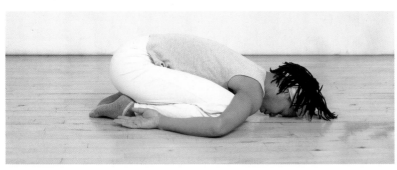

4 Counterbalance stretch Come back out of the stretch in the stages with which you went down. When you are back up, lean forward to counterbalance the stretch. Relax and breathe deeply, resting your forehead on the floor in front of you.

The Heart and Small Intestine

Heart and Small Intestine are part of the Fire element and govern the emotions. This stretch helps to bring the emotions into balance and to feel centred and calm. It opens the hips and pelvis.

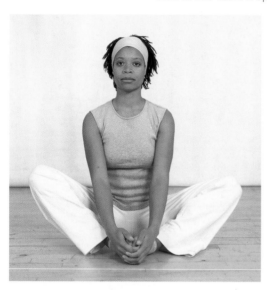 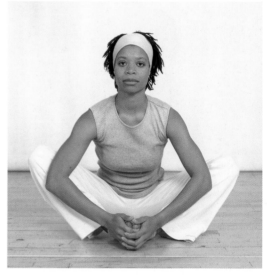

1 Feet together and face forwards Sit with your knees apart and feet soles together. Clasp your feet, keeping your back upright and your shoulders and face pointing forward.

2 Leaning forward On the out breath lean forward, bending from the hips and keeping the back straight. After 3–4 breaths relax into the stretch. Come back up on the in breath.

Heart Protector and Triple Heater

These two meridians associated with Secondary Fire have no Western equivalent. Heart Protector shields the heart and Triple Heater governs the peripheral circulation. They are responsible for a healthy and balanced emotional state.

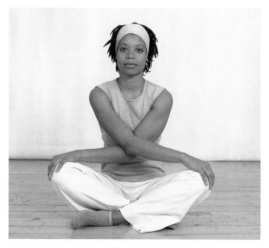

Crossing arms and legs As the photograph to the left shows, sit in cross-legged position with a straight back and cross your arms. Bring the hands on to the knees. On the out breath bend forward, keeping the back straight. Stay in this position for a couple of breaths, stretching the hands away from each other to get more of a stretch in the arms. Come back up on an in breath and repeat, crossing the arms and legs the other way round.

The Kidney and Bladder

This stretch opens up the back and activates both the Kidney and Bladder meridians. These meridians are ruled by Water, helping balance the water in your system, and can treat retention, bloatedness and dryness of the skin and hair.

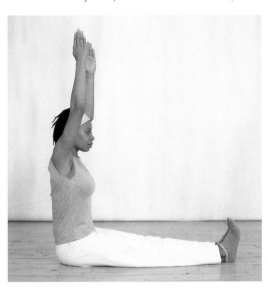

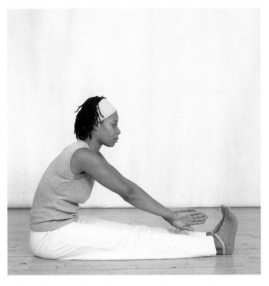

1 Bend from the hips Sit with your legs straight out in front of you. Lift your arms above your head and, breathing out, bend forward from the hips, keeping your back straight.

2 Hands between feet Bring your hands towards the feet, pushing the hands, with little fingers up, between the feet. If you can't reach your feet, hold your ankles or shins.

Gall Bladder and Liver

These meridians are associated with Wood. Gall Bladder is important in the process of decision-making and Liver governs the smooth flow of chi throughout the organs. It also provides flexibility and the ability to change direction when needed.

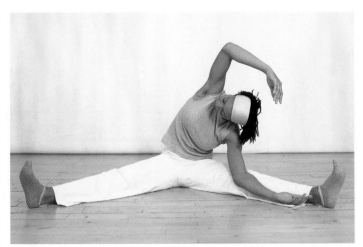

Lean over stretching your waist This exercise shows how to stretch open the meridians on the side of the body, especially affecting the Gall Bladder and Liver meridians. Sit with your legs straight and apart. Point your toes upwards and stretch your heels and ankles back, feeling the muscles in the back of your thighs as you go. Raising your arms over your head, lean your body over to one side, stretching your waist and the side of your chest. Make sure that you keep your body facing forward, and only bend sideways, not forwards.

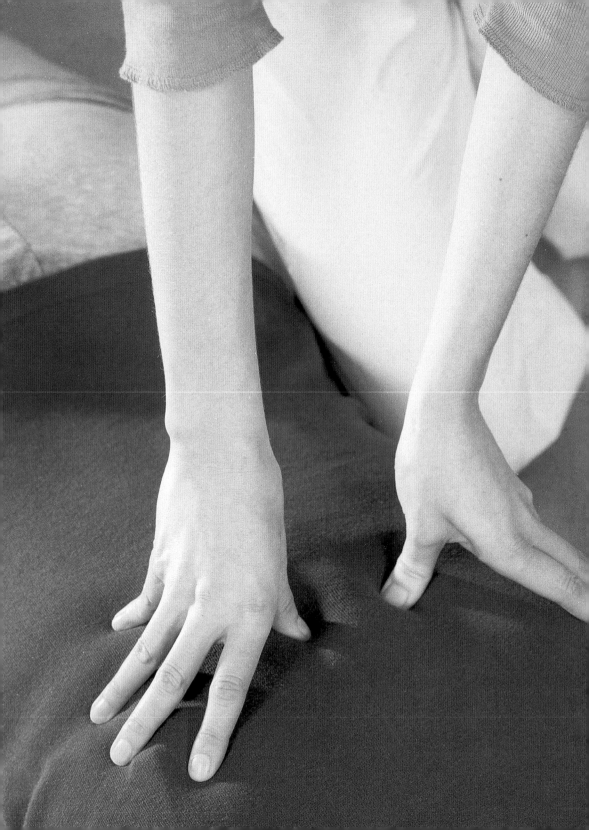

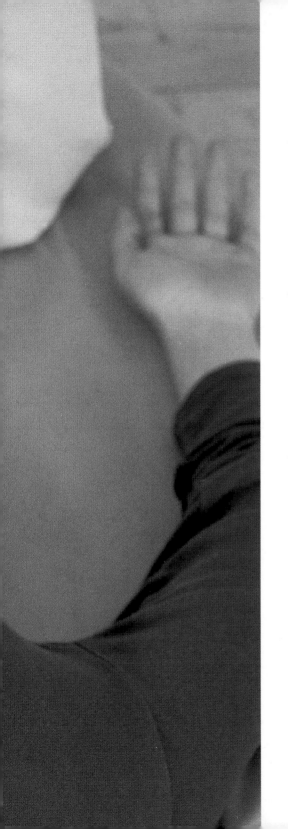

The Basic Framework

By following the step-by-step Shiatsu framework described in this chapter you can start to practise what you are learning by working on others. The framework shows a clear progression around the body, starting with the back and finishing with the feet, covering all parts in a smooth and flowing way.

This basic treatment, once mastered, can be used as a basis for designing a whole treatment, paying special attention to the appropriate meridians. If, for example, your receiver needs special attention to the back, you should proceed through the entire basic frame, but spend more time on the back. Practise this step-by-step process on any willing friends and family until you can give an entire treatment without having to think what to do next.

Preparing Yourself

Although the treatment that follows is suitable for most people, you should check with the contraindications listed on the page opposite if your receiver has any medical conditions. You also need to organize an appropriate location as well as clothing and equipment, and ensure that you are physically prepared for a session, taking particular care of your hands and fingernails. Finally, you need to prepare yourself mentally.

TREATMENT ROOM

A Shiatsu session should be performed in a warm, light room, preferably one that is simply furnished and clutter-free. Avoid using harsh or bright lights. Use a thin futon with a cover or a clean cotton sheet for the receiver to lie on, or alternatively two or three blankets covered by a sheet. You will also need some small cushions to make your partner comfortable and a blanket to cover them if they get cold or to cover them at the end of the treatment.

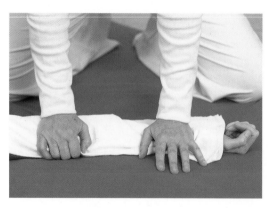

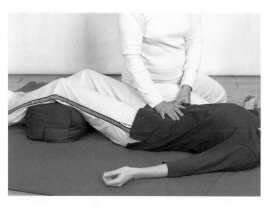

CLOTHING

Both you and your partner should wear loose, preferably cotton, trousers, top and socks so that you can both stretch and move around easily. Shiatsu is given through the clothes and it is better if your partner wears clothes with long sleeves and socks. Use a soft cotton cloth to work through where the skin is exposed. Shiatsu should not be performed on the skin.

PHYSICAL AND MENTAL PREPARATION

Make sure that your hands are clean and your fingernails are short and smooth. It is important to look after your hands regularly, because they are your Shiatsu tools. Do the preparation exercises for the hands on pages 36–7 to warm them up and increase flexibility, feeling the chi energy in your hands after you have done the exercises. If you have poor circulation or your hands are always cold, do the hand exercises every day.

How to start treatment

- Check that your partner is sitting or lying comfortably, and use supporting cushions if necessary
- Be calm, centred and sensitive, with hara breathing and a good posture, taking your time
- Focus for a few minutes, sitting quietly, meditating or exercising
- Observe your partner, noting anything that attracts your attention
- First contact should be gentle and reassuring, as you become "as one" with your partner
- Synchronize your breathing with your partner's, keeping your mind empty and receptive to your partner's energy

Above left If your partner has short sleeves, or other exposed areas of skin, lay a soft cotton cloth over the area and work through the cloth.

Left A cushion can be placed under the knees if the receiver has a stiff back. A cushion under the head or neck can help the neck and upper back.

Care and contraindications

As with every therapeutic treatment, care must be taken if one or both of the participants have medical conditions. There are some contraindications, meaning conditions in which you wouldn't give treatment, to giving Shiatsu both for giver and receiver. If you are treating someone for the first time, check down the following list beforehand:

- As a beginner, do not give a Shiatsu if your receiver has a serious condition such as cancer, a serious heart disease (although mild heart disease or angina can benefit from Shiatsu) or has had recent major surgery. If in doubt your partner should check with their doctor.
- It is also advised not to give Shiatsu to someone in the first trimester of pregnancy and there are some contraindicated points (GB 21, LI 4 and SP 6, shown on pages 89, 64 and 75) not to be used at all in pregnancy.

Do not give Shiatsu if your receiver:
- Has a high fever
- Is intoxicated or has taken non-prescribed drugs
- Has just eaten – wait two hours after meals
- Has a serious contagious disease
- Has varicose veins, broken bones or recent scar tissue – although you can work around these areas

Do not give Shiatsu if you:
- Are fatigued or upset
- Are intoxicated
- Have a serious contagious disease

Remember your level of skill and ensure that your partner knows that you are not giving orthodox medical treatment. If you find a serious problem, refer your partner to a doctor. Ensure that they understand that a healing "reaction" such as tiredness or headaches can occur as the body adjusts to a better level of health. If in doubt ask an experienced practitioner.

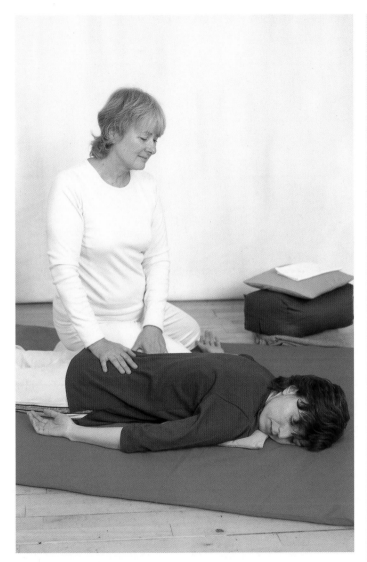

Above When the receiver is lying on his or her front, cushions can help to support the body, especially in sore or stiff areas. A cushion may be placed under the chest if the neck is stiff or the breasts are sore. Some people can feel more comfortable with a small cushion under the ankles as this relaxes the legs and feet.

Shiatsu should not be given or received by someone who has just eaten a large meal, so wait several hours before giving or receiving Shiatsu and advise your partner to do the same. This is because lying down with pressure applied to your torso after a full meal would feel uncomfortable.

Having the right frame of mind is crucial, so ensure that you relax and remain focused before you give a Shiatsu treatment.

Practise the preparation exercises outlined in the Do-in chapter (see pages 24–43) before starting your treatment; this will increase your flexibility and comfort in working around the floor.

How to Give Shiatsu

During a Shiatsu treatment it is important for both giver and receiver to remain relaxed and connected and not to overstretch the body. Here are the basic guidelines: remember them every time you give or receive Shiatsu in order to ensure a beneficial treatment. With practice it should become instinctive, so that you won't need to think about the guidelines consciously, but you may still need an occasional reminder.

RELAXATION

A comfortable physical and mental condition is essential for Shiatsu. Your whole body should be relaxed, especially hands, arms and shoulders, and your posture upright. Change your position if you feel tension in your back or shoulders. The receiver will relax more deeply when you are relaxed.

TWO-HANDED CONNECTEDNESS

Contact with the receiver's body is maintained at all times. The mother hand, or more passive hand, keeps constant contact while the other hand can move along the meridian. When contact is maintained the receiver can relax without worrying about where the practitioner is going to touch next. This is a function of the autonomic nervous system (ANS). The sympathetic mode of the ANS assesses, distinguishes and tries to work out if the touch is hostile. When connection is maintained, the ANS is able to relax into the parasympathetic mode, where healing and deep relaxation occurs.

MERIDIAN CONTINUITY

The focus of Shiatsu is to treat an entire meridian, rather than individual points or regions, and this is called meridian continuity. The aim is to bring the whole meridian back into balance by encouraging the free flow of chi, opening blockages and balancing energy.

CHI PROJECTION

You need to use chi projection throughout your Shiatsu treatments. Although we talk about pressure points and Shiatsu techniques using pressure, the practitioner will

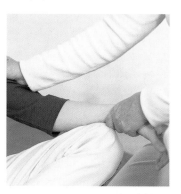

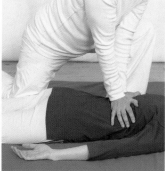

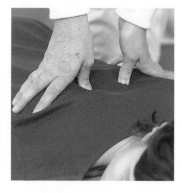

Hugging and palming Always use a hugging hand to increase relaxation by softening your hand when palming. Practise working down the arm as if you were hugging the arm with your hand. Remember how it feels to give and receive a hug, when the whole of your body softens. This is just the same feeling that you need to create when giving Shiatsu.

Body weight Position your body so you can use body weight to give pressure, rather than muscle power. Always move from your hara, using the knee-walking shown on page 31. Use a wide, stable stance, with your knees apart, to transfer your weight into the move. Keep your centre of gravity low and place yourself so that the area you are working on is in front of you and close to the hara.

Perpendicular penetration Pressure is always perpendicular, at 90 degrees to the body surface. Rather than movement across the surface, Shiatsu involves penetration at each point. Treatment involves simple, inward-directed hand movements, and not rotation, back-and-forth, or wiggling movements. Even when the body is not parallel to the ground, maintain perpendicular pressure.

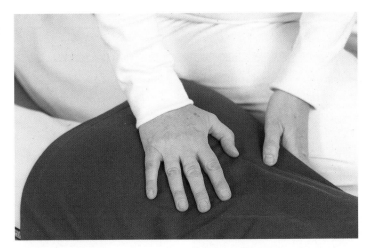

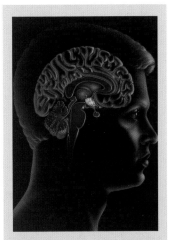

actually project his or her chi when working on a point or meridian. The result will be greater penetration, and this is an entirely different experience for the receiver than just pressing.

KYO AND JITSU

These Japanese terms, roughly meaning empty and full, are used to describe the state of energy as observed in the body. Energy can manifest in three different ways. There can be too little energy, a kyo situation, which results in a weakness or depleted function. There can be too much energy, a jitsu situation, which can manifest as tension or pain. Or energy can be stuck as a result of either fullness or emptiness. In a kyo case this will result in an empty pocket through which no energy can pass. In jitsu this is often an area of fullness that can't move anywhere, becoming stuck or stagnated. Kyo and jitsu are used to describe the quality of energy, for example a kyo area will appear lacklustre whereas jitsu may be stiff. The type of treatment required will then be based on this assessment. Generally a more kyo area will be

Kyo is empty, hidden, the cause, hollow and soft.
Jitsu is full, obvious, the effect, raised and hard.

Above There is always a mother (passive) hand (the hand on the right) and a hand that moves around the meridians (the hand on the left). Instead of the sweeping, stroking movements common to other massage techniques, Shiatsu pressure is perpendicular and uses chi projection.

Above right The hypothalamus, a control centre of the autonomic nervous system.

treated with tonifying techniques such as holding and slower, calmer work. Jitsu areas will be treated with more dispersing techniques such as rubbing, rocking and faster work, with the aim of redistributing the energy and moving blockages. In a treatment, kyo will pull you in and not resist, while jitsu will push you back out and make you bounce back. Kyo is considered to be the underlying cause of a condition and jitsu its effect. For the most effective treatment you need to look for the kyo and work with that. When the kyo is addressed, then the jitsu can relax.

GETTING FEEDBACK

Ask your partner how comfortable they feel with your pressure – they should always feel relaxed. Never overstretch or force movement so that your partner experiences pain or resistance. You may not want to keep asking for feedback, as talking could disturb them out of deep relaxation, but make it clear at the beginning that they should say if anything feels uncomfortable.

Autonomic nervous system (ANS)
The autonomic nervous system (ANS) deals with the automatic functioning of body systems, such as the digestive system, the heartbeat and water metabolism. It is the ANS that makes our organ functions start up and stop or change automatically when they are needed, without us being conscious of this happening.

There are two branches of the ANS: the sympathetic branch and the parasympathetic branch. The sympathetic branch controls the "fight and flight" mechanism, deciding when the body needs to go into action to deal with stress, by stimulating the production of adrenalin and increasing the blood supply to muscles, shutting down any unnecessary organ functions. The parasympathetic branch has the opposite function, of helping the body to relax and recuperate by slowing down the heartbeat, relaxing the muscular system, stimulating the digestion and encouraging the conservation of energy in the body.

In Shiatsu massage, the aim is to relax and calm the body, bringing the parasympathetic branch to the fore. This approach is designed to bring a deep relaxation that helps to replenish vital energies.

The Back

The back is one of the most satisfying areas of the body to treat and also to receive treatment upon. The basic routine starts with the back due to its importance in relaxing the nervous system and therefore the energy balance of the whole body.

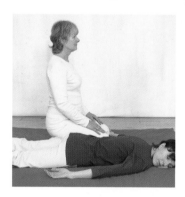

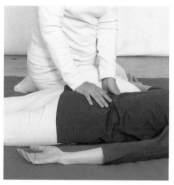

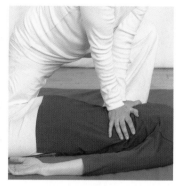

1 Prepare and breathe Start by sitting in seiza next to your partner who is in prone position (lying on their front). Sit with the outside of your leg in contact with your partner's left side. Take some deep breaths into your hara – you can close your eyes if you wish for complete concentration – and focus your attention into your hara. Open your eyes slowly and observe your partner's back.

2 Rest your hand Gently place your hand palm down on to the sacrum at the base of the spine. Be aware that this is your first contact with your partner. Notice how their body feels under your hand – it may feel hot or cold or you may feel a tingling sensation. Let your hand rest here for a couple of breaths while you "tune in to your partner". It will help if you match your breathing with your partner's.

3 Lean your weight Come into position with one knee up and one down. Starting one hand's width below the shoulders, place both palms either side of the spine and lean your body weight into your hands as you breathe out. Ask your partner to breathe out slowly with you as you apply pressure. Shift your weight back and move your hands down a little and lean in again.

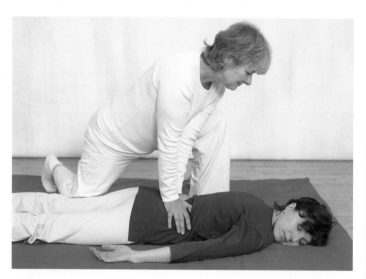

4 Move down the spine Continue down either side of the spine until you reach the sacrum, which is the base of the spine. You may have to move your legs back as you get further down the spine so that you are still comfortable and using your body weight. Check with your partner that they are comfortable with your pressure.

The sacrum
When your hand is on the sacrum, what do you feel? Do you feel hot or cold? Is there a tingling? Do you have an image? Try and find a word or a picture to describe it. Observe if some areas are looking more full or empty than others. Notice if there is a difference between the right and left sides of the body. Notice differences in the shoulders or feet or places of tension.

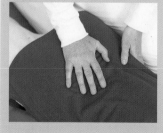

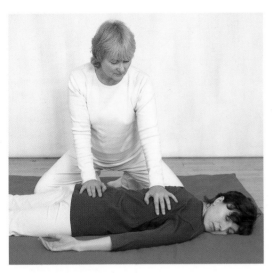

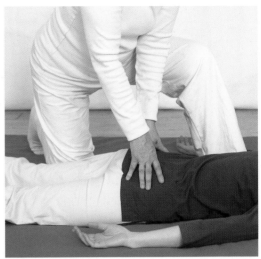

5 Rock the body Change your position so that you are facing the body from the side with both knees on the ground but wide. Place one hand on the sacrum and rock the body gently from side to side, using your body weight to maintain a rhythm. With the other hand, work down first one side of the spine then the other, maintaining the rocking rhythm with both hands and your body weight. Let the movement come to a gradual stop.

6 Lean in to apply pressure Change your position back to one knee down and one knee up (as in step 3). Starting at the top of the spine, one hand's width below the shoulders, thumb down either side of the spine on the Bladder meridian. Work with straight thumbs, two finger-widths from the midline of the spine, leaning in with your body weight to apply pressure. Work down the back slowly, moving a little way down each time.

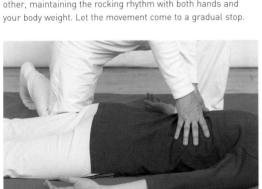

7 Move down to the sacrum
Continue to work down with your thumbs until you reach the sacrum. There are three natural depressions in the sacrum which your thumbs will fit into. Notice if there is a difference in the depth of penetration as you go down the spine. Check with your partner that they are comfortable with the pressure.

Thumb positioning
It is important to keep the thumbs straight as you work, otherwise you will put strain on the joints of your thumbs.

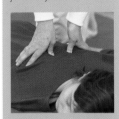

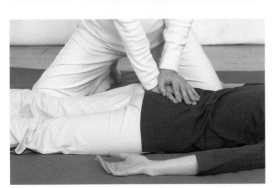

8 Sustain pressure and breathe Place both hands on the sacrum and lean in. Stay in that position while you and your partner breathe in and out slowly a few times, and then gradually ease the pressure. Come back to position 1, with your hand on the sacrum. Notice if there has been a change in the feeling under your hand.

Use your other fingers to provide support for your thumbs. Make sure your pressure is perpendicular to the body. The pressure will be more precise and directed, and the energy will come directly from your hara and into the receiver.

The Legs and Buttocks

As you work on the backs of the legs you will be accessing the rest of Bladder meridian, the longest meridian in the body. The buttocks are important in boosting energy to the reproductive system. There are some sensitive points in this area.

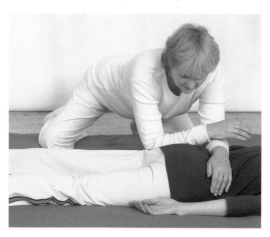

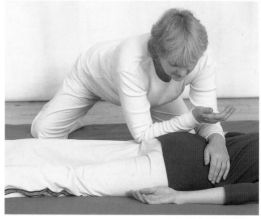

1 Forearm on buttocks Face your partner's body from the side with both knees on the ground but wide apart. Lean forwards so that you can comfortably work with your forearm on the buttocks. Start with your left forearm on the sacrum as the mother arm. Beginning at the side of the buttock nearest you, bending your elbow, place your right forearm gently on to the buttock, and roll your right arm away from you over the buttock and back.

2 Repeat the rolling motion Do this over the whole of the left buttock, altering your position if necessary in order to cover the whole area. Make sure that you are using the weight of your body as pressure, without putting too much pressure into the mother arm resting on the sacrum. Feel the energy coming from your hara, lowering your hara towards the ground for greater stability if necessary by adopting a wider kneeling position.

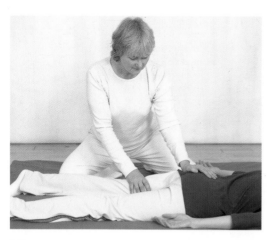

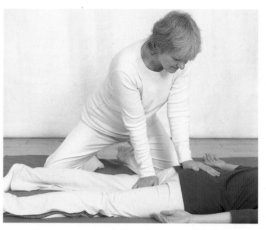

3 Sit up slightly and work your hand down the leg nearest you With the mother hand still on the sacrum, squeeze and knead down the leg to the ankle, using each squeeze to rock the leg gently and promote the movement of energy. If the knees are painful on the floor, place a small cushion under the calves.

4 Apply energy from your hara Come back up to the top of the leg and, keeping the left hand on the sacrum, palm down the back of the leg to the ankle. Use your body weight to apply energy, and feel it coming from your hara. Do not press on the back of the knee and go straight on to the lower leg.

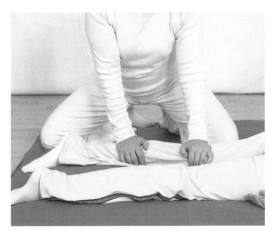

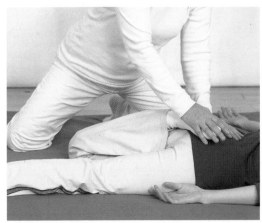

5 Break contact with sacrum If your partner has long legs you may need to move your mother hand to just above the knee so that you can reach right down to their ankles. Holding the leg below the knee, break contact with the sacrum and gently place it a hand's width above the knee, without increasing the pressure.

6 Stretch the foot Pick up the foot with one hand under the ankle, keeping your other hand on the sacrum. Stretch the foot to the buttock above this leg. You can push the top of the foot down so that the front of the ankle is opened, but be careful not to overstretch. Check with your partner for comfort.

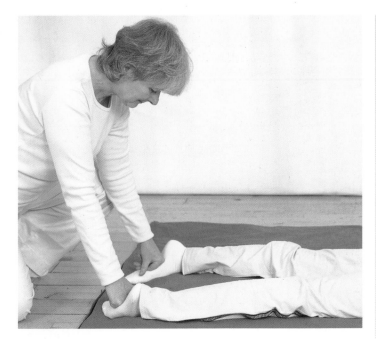

7 Pressure on soles and arches Come to the base of the feet and apply pressure to the soles and arches with your knuckles, without clenching your thumb into your hand. Lean in, putting your weight into your knuckles. To treat the other leg move to the other side and pick up the leg under the ankle and stretch it towards the buttock as in step 6. Change position so that you are at the top of the leg. Repeat steps 1–4 on the leg, using your other hand to work across the buttocks and down the leg. While you are moving, keep one hand as a mother hand connected to the body at all times.

Cushions

If you notice that your partner is not able to fully relax or that parts of the body do not make contact with the floor, this can show you where there are areas of stiffness and tension. When applying pressure use cushions to support any stiff or painful joints. For example, if someone has tight ankles or has had an ankle injury, you may notice that the shin is not touching the floor. Place a cushion under the shin so that as you apply pressure you will not put undue strain on the ankle joint. You can then safely let your weight drop on to the back of the leg. Similarly a cushion under the shin can protect a problem knee.

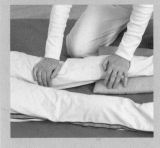

The Front and the Hara

Ask your partner to turn over on to their back, into the supine position. Make sure
they are comfortable, with the back and back of the legs in contact with the floor.
Place a cushion under the knees if the lower back is uncomfortable.

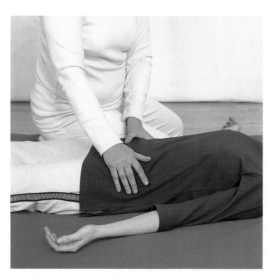

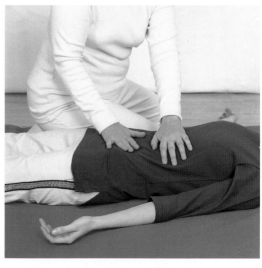

1 Hands on waist Sit in seiza next to your partner on the right
and place your hands either side of the waist, slightly to the front.
Keep the pressure gentle as this is a vulnerable area.

2 Feel the outline of the hara The ribs make the upper border,
and the hip bones create the lower border. The navel will be on
the waist level, slightly above the centre of the hara.

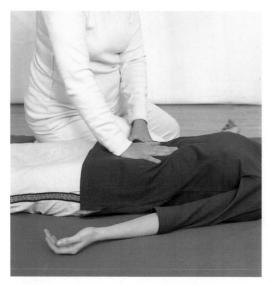

Gentle pressure

Remember that this is a very vulnerable area of the body,
so pressure should be light to begin with. Check with your
partner if your pressure is comfortable. Tune in to their
energy. Observe any sensations under your hand. If
someone is ticklish make your contact firm and confident,
and if all fails, come back to the hara later in the session.

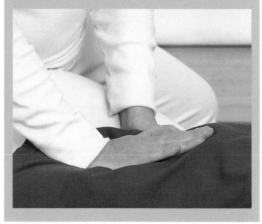

3 Slide your right hand gently to the centre of the hara
Do this with your palm resting just below the navel and your
fingers spread over it, but not reaching the base of the ribs.
Keep the left hand at the side of the waist as the mother hand.

4 Create a wave-like motion Place your right hand on the hara with your fingers pointing towards the head, and the heel of your hand just above the pubic bone. Press the heel of your hand down with the out breath and release on the in breath, pushing the fingers down, making a wave-like motion from the heel of the hand to the fingertips. Keep the pressure soft and flowing, without any abrupt or jerky movements. Ask your partner to breathe in and out with your pressure, and keep the rhythm of the movement steady and flowing, following the breath.

5 Stroke around the hara Do this with a light clockwise movement using both hands. This is a very relaxing movement that will focus the energy of your partner into the hara. Ask your partner to breathe slowly in and out, concentrating the breath into the hara and imagining it glowing with every in breath.

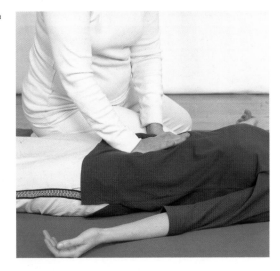

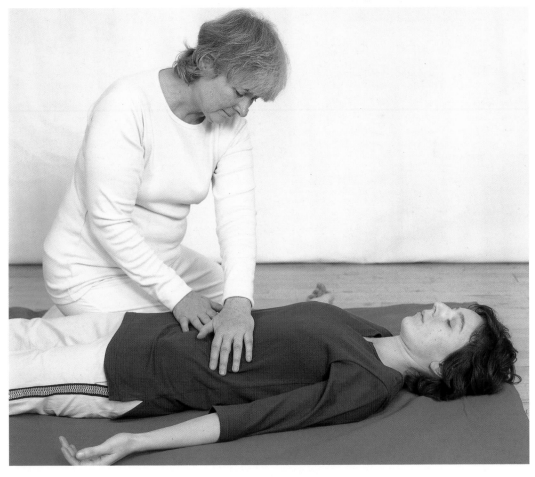

The Arms

There are six meridian pathways beginning and ending at the fingertips and flowing through the arms, some continuing into the shoulders and neck. This sequence stretching and palming the arms will help to increase chi flow into all these areas.

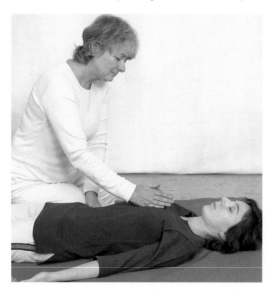

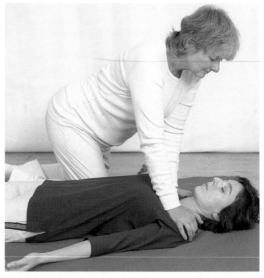

1 Work up the sternum Kneel comfortably on the right of your partner, the end of your knees about level with their elbow. Place your left hand on the side of the body as the mother hand. From the centre of the hara, using the little finger side of your right hand, work up the sternum to the left shoulder.

2 Stretch open the shoulders Change position to one knee forward and the other back. Bringing your hand on to the right shoulder, lean in with your body weight to stretch open the shoulders. Make a mental note of any tension or difference in the shoulders. Does one go down easier than the other?

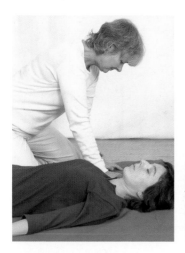

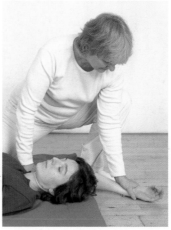

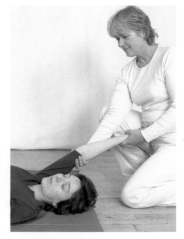

3 Palm down With the mother hand (now the right hand) on the right shoulder, bring the arm out at 90 degrees and palm down from the shoulder towards the hand.

4 Lift and stretch Lift the arm by the wrist and stretch it up over the head. Only stretch it up as far as it will move easily, without strain.

5 Arm off ground Move to the top of the head, lifting the arm up off the ground. Lean back and stretch the arm from the shoulder, supporting the elbow and wrist.

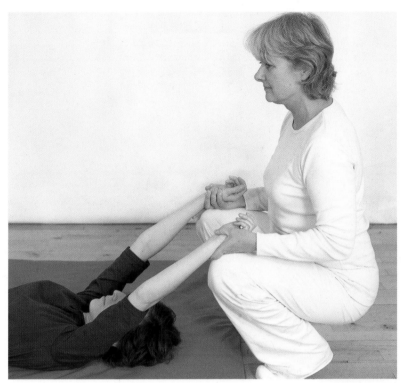

6 Stretch both arms Keeping hold of the right arm, lift the other above the head. In squatting position, lean back and stretch both arms. Be careful when stretching, holding the arms at the wrists with a soft hold. Never extend a stretch beyond your partner's natural extent, and be extra cautious on areas of the body that have previously been injured or are problematic.

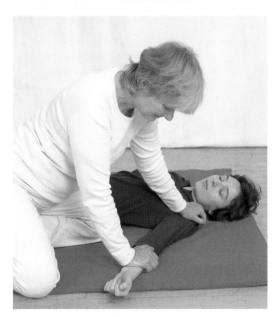

7 Palm down Let go of the right hand, move round so that the left arm is now at 90 degrees and palm down this arm.

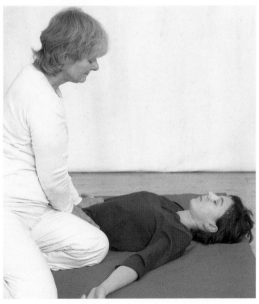

8 Rest gently Sit back in seiza at the hara and let your hand rest gently on the hara. Notice changes from the start of the exercise.

The Legs

As you work on the legs, notice any differences in the right and left sides: is one side easier to work than the other, or lighter and more flexible? The extent of the natural turn-out of the feet when lying down will be linked to the tension in the hip.

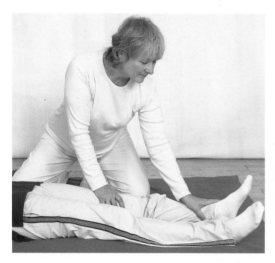

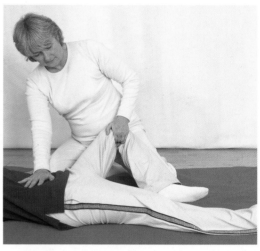

1 Palm down With your partner lying on their back, sit in seiza on the left side. Palm down the outside of the left leg, with your mother hand moving from the hara to above the knee if necessary.

2 Pick up the leg With your mother hand on the hara, pick up the leg by placing your left hand under the knee and bringing it towards you. Move your hand to the front of the bent knee, and bring it back to vertical, then up towards your partner's head.

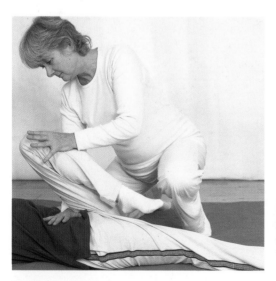

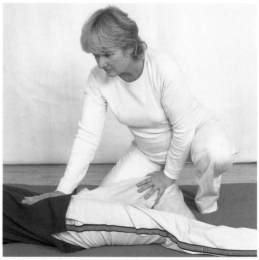

3 Rotate leg outwards As you bring up the leg, change your position to one knee up, and rotate the leg outwards to follow the natural movement of the hip joint. Keep your hand on the hara. Ask your partner to let you know if you are stretching too far. Notice any stiffness in the hip as you rotate.

4 Stretch and support Bring the leg down and, still bent, let it drop out to the side. Place the instep against the opposite knee and stretch by applying gentle pressure to the left knee towards the floor. If the bent leg does not reach the floor, support the leg with your thigh wedged under your partner's thigh.

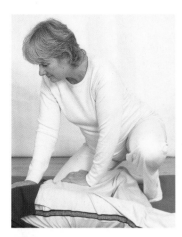

5 Palm up the leg With your hand still on the hara, palm up the inside of the leg, from above the ankle along the inside of the calf and thigh. Balance the pressure of your working hand with your mother hand. Remember to use perpendicular pressure and notice any areas of stiffness or emptiness.

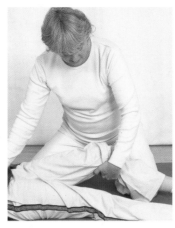

6 Gently straighten the leg Supporting the leg under the knee, return it to its original position. When you lift or bend the legs and when you ease them back down again, always do so by supporting under the knee. Take extra care if your partner has knee problems.

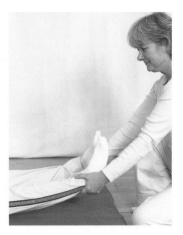

7 Lift feet off the floor Move your position to below the feet, kneeling on one knee. Take both ankles in your hands and slowly lift them off the floor with your arms straight. Stretch both legs by using your body weight to lean backwards, opening up and stretching the legs from the abdomen.

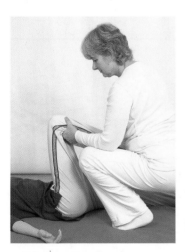

8 Transition Step to the other side of the body. Place your left hand beneath the knee and the right hand beneath the ankle of the right leg and lift the leg off the floor. As you step forward bend your partner's knee up, changing the position of your left hand to the front of the knee and the right hand to support the foot. Slide your lower leg forward so that you are in a position to rotate the leg. This should be a flowing movement.

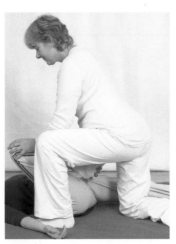

9 Rotate the leg Note the two different kinds of leg rotations: in the first rotation your hand is on the hara so that you can monitor the ease of movement of the hip; while in the second you may be able to make a bigger range of movement, useful if your partner has heavy legs, or has difficulty in letting go. Repeat steps 4–6 on this leg, ensuring that you are not over-stretching or forcing. Come back to the hara on this side.

Positions for giving Shiatsu
Many practitioners find it comfortable to sit with the legs wide apart and both knees on the floor. You will have to maintain this posture for some time, so it is important that you do not tense or strain your own spine. The knees can be brought up or down so that you can move around easily, stretch over the body, and sink your weight properly into your hara when necessary.

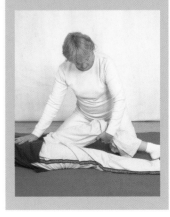

The Neck and Shoulders

The neck and shoulders are often an area of tension and discomfort. This short sequence can be done as a stand-alone treatment or incorporated into the basic treatment. Releasing tension in the neck and shoulders can increase blood flow to the head and improve alertness.

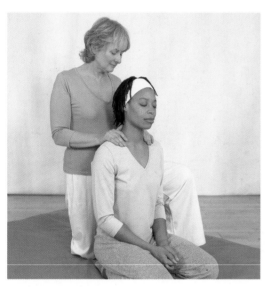

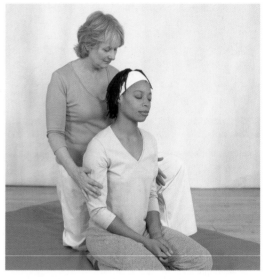

1 Tune in to your partner's energy With your partner sitting in seiza (or cross legged if this is more comfortable) kneel behind your partner, placing your hands on the shoulders.

2 Palm across the shoulders and down the arms Use a hugging hand to work down the arms to the elbows. Repeat two or three times to loosen the arms and shoulders.

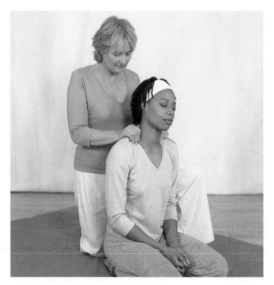

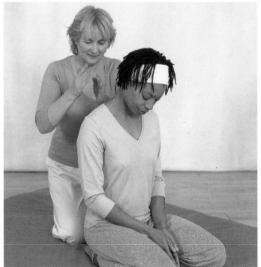

3 Squeeze the shoulders Do this by holding the trapezius muscles that run along the top of the shoulders and into the back of the neck. Try shaking, rocking, and kneading with the squeeze.

4 Light taps With your hands straight but relaxed and the sides of your hands towards your partner, cover the shoulder and upper back area with rapid, light taps.

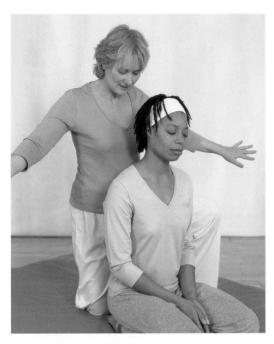

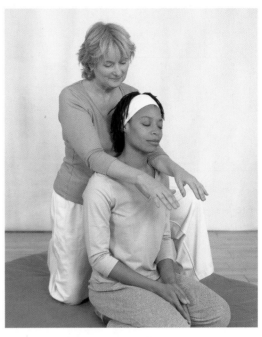

5 Brush hands out In one great sweeping motion, sweep your hands from the top of the shoulders, brushing them out.

6 Pressure down Balance your forearms on the shoulders of your partner, next to the neck, and gently put pressure down.

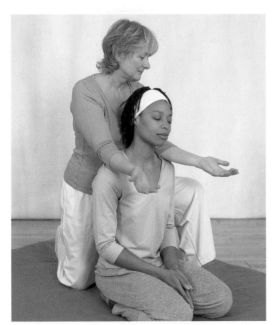

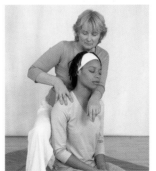

8 Press with thumb Leaving one of your arms on your partner's shoulder, press along the top of the shoulder with your thumb. Repeat on other shoulder.

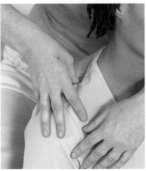

9 Focus on pressure point Work in to the pressure point GB 21, situated on the top of the trapezius muscle midway between the base of the neck and the end of the shoulder. This is a good point for releasing tension in the shoulder. Do not work on this point during pregnancy.

7 Rolling on shoulders and turning palms Roll your forearms along the tops of your partner's shoulders, turning the palms of your hands upwards.

▷

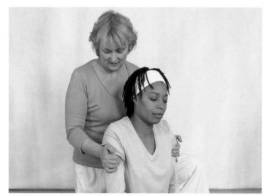

10 Shoulders in shrug Holding the top of the arms, lift up the shoulders into a shrug to see if the shoulders are relaxed.

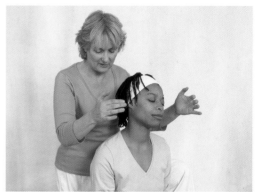

11 Release the shoulders Having done this, the shoulders should return to their natural position. Repeat a few times.

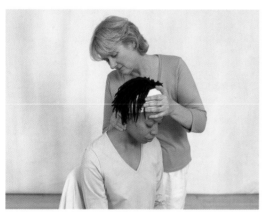

12 Drop head Holding the front of the head, let it drop forward. Squeeze down the back of the neck either side of the spine.

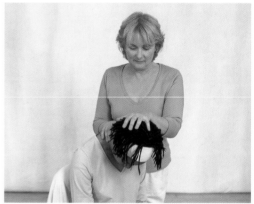

13 Hold stretch Let the head drop forwards gently, taking care not to overstretch. Hold the stretch for a few seconds.

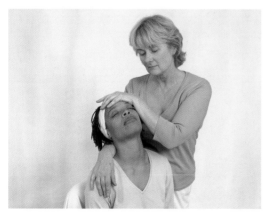

14 Drop head back Do this holding the forehead with one hand and with your other forearm behind the neck for support.

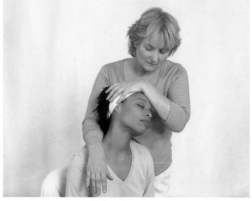

15 Head towards you Holding the side of the head, bend it to the side towards you, with your arm on the opposite shoulder.

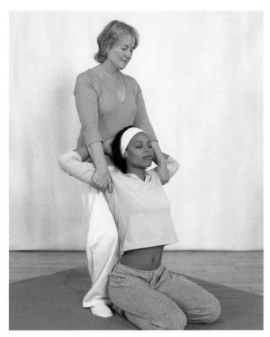

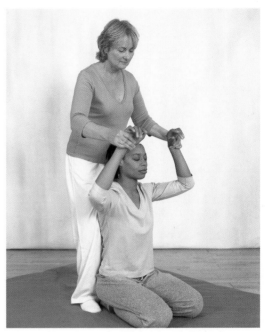

16 Stretch arms Stand with your knees against your partner and ask them to clasp their hands behind their head. Reaching under the arms, stretch up and back.

17 Hold arms Taking your partner's arms up by the wrists, hold them gently above the head, checking they are relaxed.

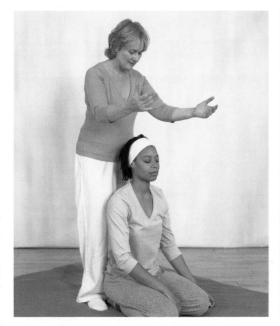

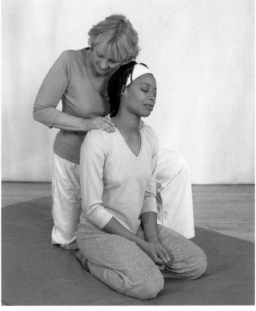

18 Let arms drop Release your hold and let your partner's arms drop naturally back into place, falling on to the lap.

19 Tune in Kneel down again, place your palms back on your partner's shoulders and tune in. Notice any changes.

The Hands

The hands are worked in a similar way to that described in the Do-in section. There are many important meridian points on both hands and feet. Include this sequence into the basic routine when working on the arms.

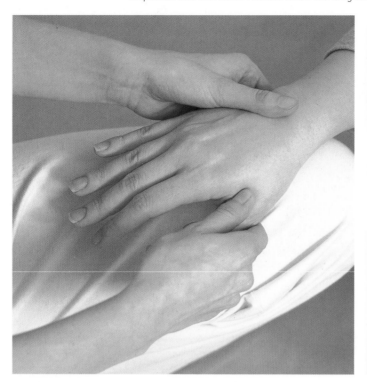

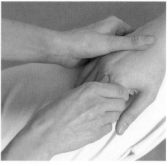

2 Massage fingers Massage thumbs and fingers, squeezing along each.

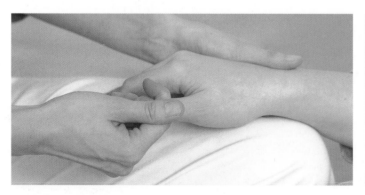

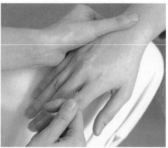

3 Stretch Holding the wrist, gently pull each finger and the thumb.

1 Rotate and flick Holding your partner's hand, rotate the thumb and fingers both ways, and then flick them one by one.

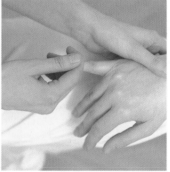

4 Find the point LI 4 This pressure point is located in the depression where the two bones of the thumb and index finger meet. Press in with your thumb towards the bone of the index finger and hold. This point is good for constipation or diarrhoea and is known as "the great eliminator". Do not use in pregnancy.

5 Squeeze fingertips Squeeze the sides at the base of the fingernails – this stimulates the finishing points of the arm meridians.

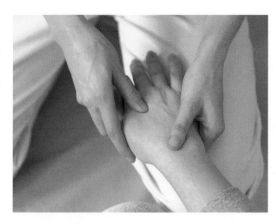

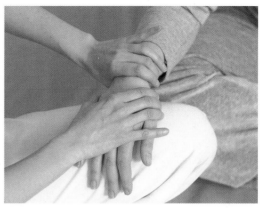

6 Fingers to wrist Holding with one hand, work with your thumb between the metacarpals from the fingers to the wrist.

7 Encircle wrist and twist Rotate the wrists by encircling the upper and lower wrist and gently twisting to either side.

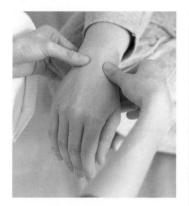

8 Shake hand Holding wrists between the thumb and forefingers, shake the hand up and down to relax the wrist.

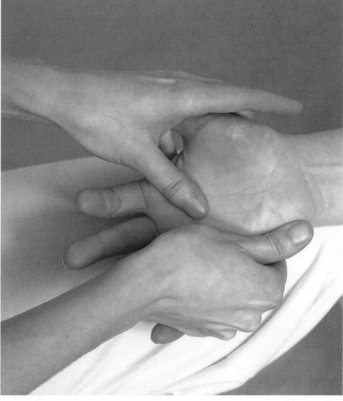

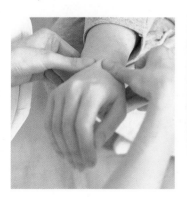

9 Work the wrists Use your thumbs to work the wrists, easing between the bones of the wrist on the front and back.

10 Open the palm With your partner's palm up, open up the palm by slotting your little fingers between the thumb and forefinger and the little finger and fourth finger. Stretch open the palm and use your thumbs to massage into the palm. Find HP 8 in the centre of the palm – fold the fingers down and it is where the middle finger touches the palm – and massage with your thumb. Repeat the full sequence on the other hand.

The Feet

There are many key points in the feet meridians, which you can include when giving a complete treatment. Finishing a treatment with the feet is a nice way to ground the energy. Shiatsu on the feet should be given through clean, preferably cotton socks.

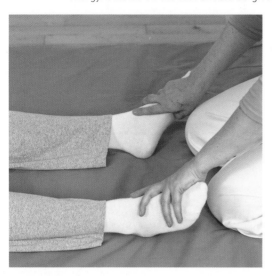

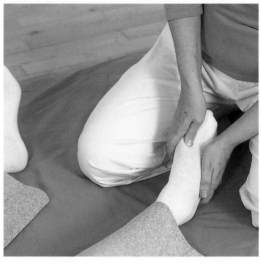

1 Bubbling spring Find KD 1 on the sole of the feet where the pad of the big toe and the ball of the foot make a "V", about a third of the way from the middle toe to the heel (see page 82). This "Bubbling Spring" point is a revitalizing point.

2 Open up foot Working on the top of the foot, use the side of your thumb and the heel of the other hand to work into the top of the foot from the middle to the edges, squeezing and pressing towards the outside edge.

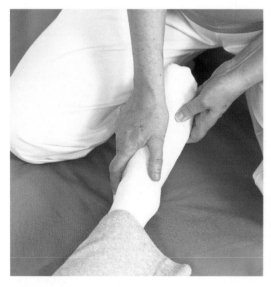

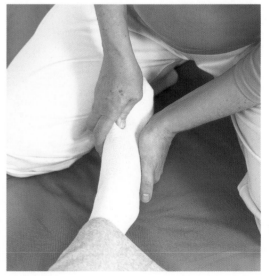

3 Open up sole of foot Squeeze the feet between your palms, grasping the sides of the feet and opening up the sole of the foot like a book. Work from the toes towards the heel a couple of times.

4 Work into the bones Work in between the metatarsals (the bones of the foot which become the toes) with your thumb. Be aware that there are some painful points here.

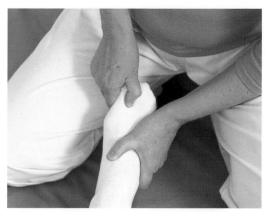

5 Unblock Liver energy Find LV 3, between the big toe and the second toe, two finger-widths below the webbing.

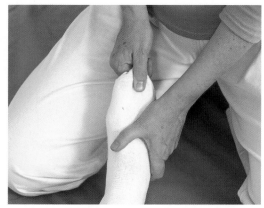

6 Massage, rotate and flick Do this to each toe to stimulate the meridians. Pinch between each of the toes.

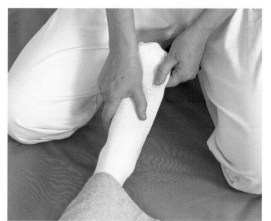

7 Hold and pull Holding the foot with the other hand, hold each toe, gently pulling to straighten it.

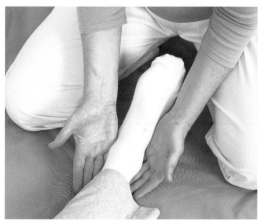

8 Rub around the ankle Do this with the sides of your hands, moving your hands firmly over the whole area.

9 Achilles tendon With fingers and thumb, squeeze down either side of the Achilles tendon. Find KD 3 on the inside of the ankle between the Achilles tendon and the tip of the ankle bone. This point is good for lower back pain.

Repeat the whole exercise on the other foot.

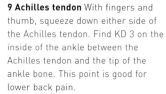

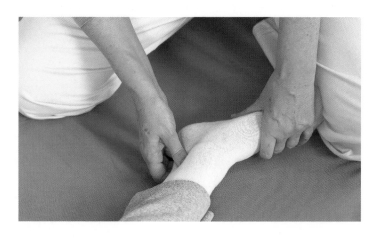

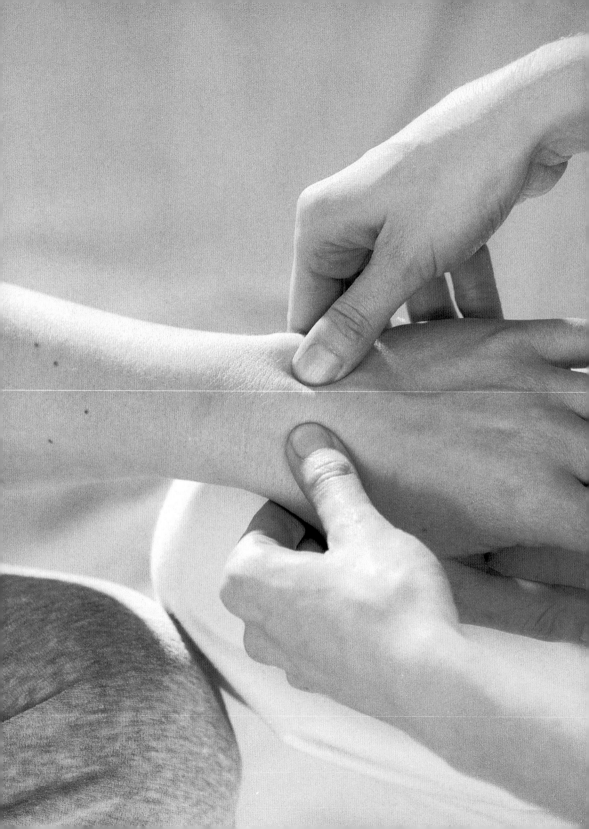

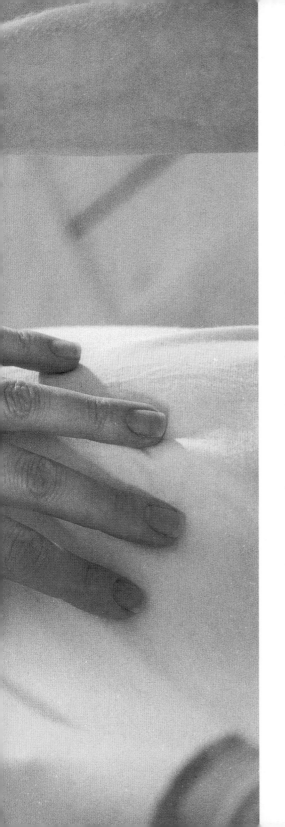

The Elements and Meridians

Here we look at the general nature of the five elements – Earth, Metal, Water, Wood and Fire (which breaks down into Primary Fire and Secondary Fire). Exploring the connection between the characteristics of each element and its associated pair of meridians, a series of Shiatsu sequences are then introduced, designed to work on each of the meridian pathways.

Although the meridians have, in most cases, the same name as a major organ in the body, their function does not necessarily correspond to the Western view of that organ. The Traditional Chinese Medicine practitioner takes a much wider view of the organ functions, ranging from emotional and psychological influences to the colour and sounds associated with the organ.

The Shiatsu treatments shown here can be used to rebalance the element in question, or used as part of a more general Shiatsu workout.

Working the Meridians

Each of the five elements has two meridians that control specific functions and body parts. In Shiatsu you can work these meridians to improve the general healthy function of the body, or to treat problems related to an element or a meridian. For simplicity, this section shows how to treat the parts of these meridians on the leg or the arm, clearly showing the first and last points of the meridian and some landmark points along each one.

PREPARATION

Before you start a treatment, do some preparation work (see preceding chapters), especially massaging and bringing energy to your hands. Also reread the contraindications section on page 47 and check that the receiver does not have any conditions that would make treatment inadvisable. Always listen to your partner's feedback. If they say that something is painful, slow down or stop what you are doing. And finally if someone has a serious complaint do not treat them. Shiatsu is not a medical treatment and should never be used as such. If you are in doubt about someone's condition refer them either to another practitioner or to a doctor.

GENERAL POSITIONS FOR MERIDIAN WORK

When treating your partner, always put the leg or arm in the position that will give you the easiest way of treating the meridian. Keep a steady rhythm going as you move along the meridian finding the landmark points. You may have to change your position slightly when you find the end points on the hands or feet.

Let the mother hand rest on the body while palming or working the points with the other hand. This hand keeps a constant pressure and gives a sense of security to the receiver, leaving the other hand free to move from point to point along the meridian. The pictures shown throughout this chapter will give you an indication of where the mother hand should be, but you can sometimes adapt the position if it is uncomfortable or hard to reach. Remember to relax, using your body weight and perpendicular pressure as you go into the meridian.

RESPONSIVENESS

As you work on your partner, go in slowly until you feel a resistance and then wait. Be aware of how the area under your hand or thumb feels. Sometimes the resistance will melt and you will be able to go further. Never force pressure on your partner: take your time and don't rush. Check with your partner if the pressure feels all right: if there is pain use less pressure or go in more slowly, or move on to a different part of the body and return to the tender part later.

As you practise you may be able to get a sense of how different areas or points on the meridian feel. Sometimes under-energized or over-energized points can be felt as a softness or stiffness, a fullness or emptiness.

INTEGRATING MERIDIAN WORK

Having practised working the individual meridians, then use the basic framework (see pages 44–67) and slot one or two meridian sequences into it. For example, while

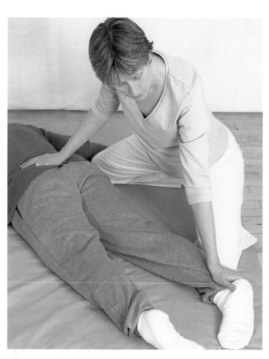

Left Use a wide seiza stance and apply pressure through your own body weight, originating from your hara.

Palming and thumbing the meridians

Palm the meridian to get a feel for where it is and the quality of the energy you are feeling (below). Then work down the points with your thumb, finding the beginning point, gradually moving along the meridian and then finding the landmark points. Keep your thumb straight when treating points, supporting it by making a fist with the fingers (below).

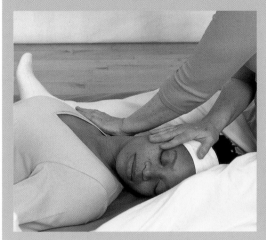

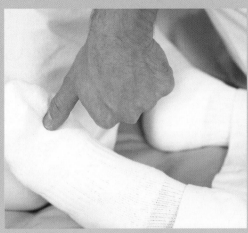

treating the legs in supine put the leg into position for Spleen meridian and work this meridian (see pages 74–5). Work all the meridian and points on one leg and then work the other side, using the transition in the basic framework outline. If you are treating two meridians on the leg, for example, treat both meridians on one leg first before moving around the body to start work on the other leg.

MERIDIANS AND ASSOCIATED PROBLEMS

Remember the first touch in the basic framework outline and use the time while your hand is resting on the sacrum to scan the body looking for areas of tension or lack of energy. Which meridians pass through these areas? If your partner reports an area of tension or a particular pain, match the area to a meridian or point.

Usually in a treatment the practitioner will treat only two or three meridians appropriate to that person's condition. Start to think about which meridians would help with specific problems when reading the section describing the characteristics of each of the five elements. For someone with digestive problems, for example, the best meridians to work could be Spleen and Stomach; for someone with a cough you could work on Lung meridian. In the next section there is a more detailed account of diagnostic skills and how to choose which meridians to work on (see pages 104–11).

Right A model showing some of the key pressure points in Traditional Chinese Medicine on the human torso.

Use your powers of observation to see how the body is responding. Sense what is going on under your hand or thumb and ask your partner for feedback. Using observation and feedback are ways of improving and developing your intuition – a combination of knowledge, observation and an ability to "listen" (hearing sounds, but also sensing, feeling and responding to the subtle signals you pick up).

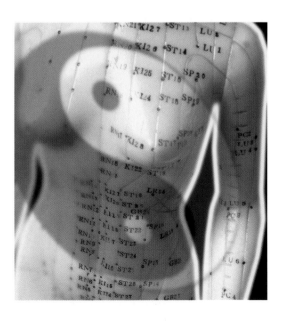

Earth

Earth represents solidity, nurturing and support, and is dependable and constant. It is associated with fertility, the cycles of nature and the reproduction of life. It provides us with food and gives us the ground beneath our feet, providing a home that grows and renews itself to support our existence. Earth's associated meridian pair is Spleen and Stomach: Spleen is the yin meridian and Stomach is the yang meridian.

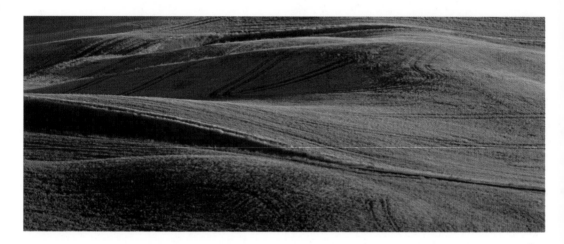

This element creates energy for digestion and governs the flesh. Earth's influence is felt throughout the front of the body, bringing energy and tone to the front muscles, especially the abdominal muscles.

When Earth is in balance a person is grounded, centred, and has the capacity to be still. The individual is then in a position to provide comfort because they feel secure and supported. The digestion is good and the appetite is stable.

Anxiety, worry and over-thinking damage Earth, knotting the energy and causing blockages in flow. Imbalance in Earth can result in digestive problems, diarrhoea, eating disorders, weight problems and menstrual problems. Someone out of balance in Earth will feel insecure, jealous or may have a victim mentality.

The most active time of day for Earth energy is 7–11a.m. This is the best time to digest food. If you hate getting up in the morning you may be out of balance in Earth. The time of year relating to Earth is late summer, and ill-health around this time could be a result of disharmony in this element. The taste attraction for Earth is sweet, especially the slow releasing, balanced

Above and below Mother Earth provides plentifully for us, bringing us nourishment, and providing stability and fertility.

sweetness of grains and root vegetables. The intense, fast-release sweetness of refined sugar will damage Earth. A craving for sweets and sugary food and drink shows a disharmony in the Stomach and Spleen meridians, indicating Earth element problems.

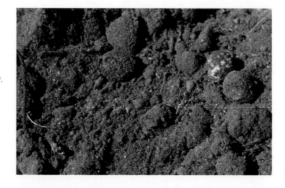

Pathway of the Stomach Meridian

Stomach meridian runs down the front of the body either side of the mouth,
through the breast and either side of the stomach. Indigestion, nausea and vomiting
can be helped by treating Stomach meridian, as well as eating disorders.

The Stomach meridian starts under the eye and runs past the side of the mouth, down the neck, crosses the collarbone and passes through the nipple. It then turns inwards at the belly and runs two finger-widths either side of the midline, branching out to the outside of the thigh. It follows the outside border of the thigh and proceeds down the outside edge of the tibia (the shin bone). It then passes on to the front of the foot and finishes at the inside corner of the toenail of the second toe, where it meets the big toe.

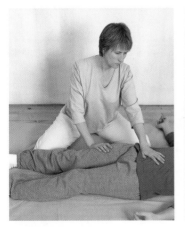

1 Turn leg inwards With your mother hand on the hara, place your lower knee against the lower leg, your hand on the thigh, and turn the leg inwards.

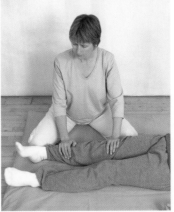

2 Palm down Keeping your hand on the hara, palm down the leg from the thigh to the ankle, changing the position of your mother hand to just above the knee.

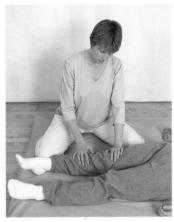

3 Thumb down Thumb down the meridian, moving the mother hand to just above the knee for the lower leg. Shift your position downwards as you go.

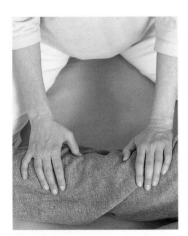

4 Find the point ST 36 This is situated three finger-widths below the knee on the outside of the leg. This is a good point for knee problems and tired legs.

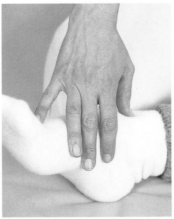

5 Find the point ST 41 This is on the front of the foot at the ankle crease between the two tendons. Use this point to help indigestion and nausea.

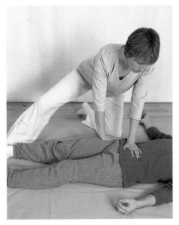

6 Foot against foot As an alternative position, you can use your foot against your partner's foot to turn the leg inward into Stomach position.

Pathway of the Spleen Meridian

Spleen helps in the digestive process by transforming food into energy and transporting this "food chi" and other fluids around the body. Treating it can help tiredness and digestive problems, such as diarrhoea and irritable bowel syndrome.

The Spleen meridian starts at the inside edge of the big toe, at the base of the toe nail. It passes along the centre of the top of the foot, and up in front of the ankle bone. As it runs up the leg, it remains along the inside edge of the tibia bone to the front, on the fleshy part. The meridian then runs along the inside edge of the

thigh muscle, passing through the centre of the groin. It then pursues a course up through the front of the belly, a hand's width either side of the body's midline. It branches outwards at the ribs, continuing around the outside edge of the breast as far as the second rib, turning down to finish just below the armpit.

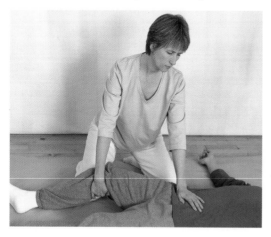

1 Face the hara Sit in seiza on the right side of your partner with your left hand on the hara. Turn to face the hara, keeping your hand on the hara as a mother hand.

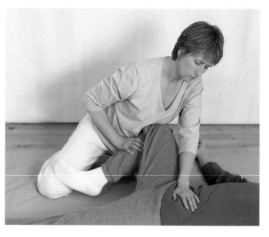

2 Leg towards you Bring up the right leg with your right hand under the knee, sliding it towards you. Change your hand to the front of the bent knee and press the leg up and sideways.

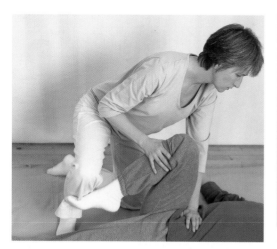

3 Rotate leg As you bring up the leg, change your position to one knee up, the other down and rotate the leg in a wide rotation. Feel for stiffness and check that it is comfortable.

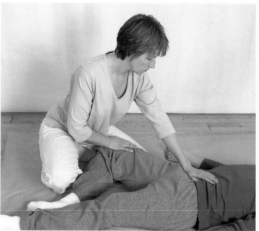

4 Lower leg down Lower the leg gently back down to the floor, with the knee bent and the heel lying just above the other ankle. Keep your hand on the hara.

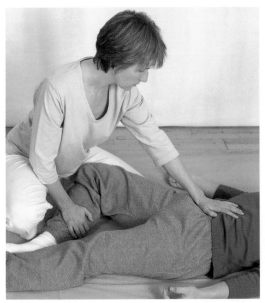

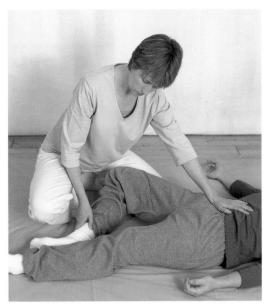

5 Palm inside leg Palm up the leg on the Spleen meridian pathway, up the inside of the leg, towards the front. Use your body weight, shifting your position when necessary.

6 Thumb pressure Use your thumb to press up the meridian. Keep your mother hand on the hara as you go, and once again move as necessary. Feel for kyo and jitsu as you work.

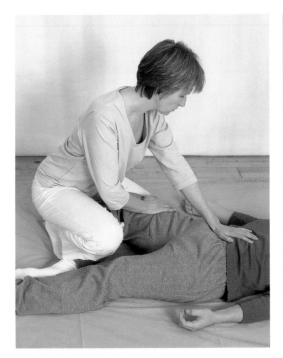

7 Turn to face the head When working on the thigh you can turn to face the head, swivelling slightly to be in position.

Spleen meridian points

Two important points on Spleen meridian are SP 6 and SP 9. SP 6 influences the digestive system, hormonal disorders and immune disorders. SP 9 is used to treat urinary diseases, abdominal and back pain and female reproductive system disorders.

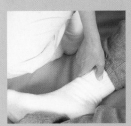

SP 6
Find this point by placing your first three fingers above the ankle bone on the inside of the leg. This point is helpful for menstrual pain and is also good for diarrhoea. Do not use during pregnancy.

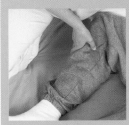

SP 9
This point is at the top of the shin bone on the inside leg in the fleshy part. It can help with knee problems, especially if the knee is swollen or is recovering from injury or surgery.

Metal

Metal is the densest of the elements, often aligned with rock and minerals. It is the force of gravity, the power of magnetism, the minerals within the earth – the rocks, the gems of the earth, the concentration of finely tuned particles. Metal is associated with strength, force, structure and boundaries. Metal's meridian pair is Lung and Large Intestine: Lung is the yin meridian and Large Intestine is the yang meridian.

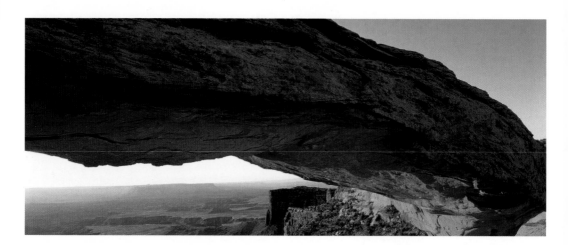

Metal governs the intake of chi and breath, inspiration and expiration. Chi from the air is transformed into what is called "true chi" and spreads throughout the body. The first of the Metal meridians, Lung sends "defensive chi" around the body, making the first line of defence against what the Chinese call "external pathogens" and what we know as infectious diseases, particularly colds and flu. If the Lung energy is weak there can be a susceptibility to diseases such as colds and coughs. Excess grief damages Lung. The second meridian, the Large Intestine, eliminates the waste products of the body.

Metal is to do with communication, boundaries, and taking in and letting go. The skin is the tissue associated with Metal. The skin makes the boundary of our bodies but it is not rigid. It is a permeable, living, breathing organ. The Lungs and Large Intestine act as boundaries which control the passage of substances in and out of the body.

People with a healthy Lung and Large Intestine function are open with a positive attitude. Good communicators, they have an ability to let go when needed but maintain boundaries when necessary. They will have healthy eliminations, a strong voice and be resistant to disease.

Above Rocks are symbolic of the Metal element in the environment (see also below), forming a cold, solid structure.

People with an imbalance in Metal can be either rigid and unable to let go or the opposite, having no boundaries. They will have a susceptibility to excessive colds and coughs and respiratory disease. Skin problems and constipation can be a sign of Metal imbalance. The taste attraction for Metal is pungent or spicy, but excess spicy food can cause Large Intestine problems. The season when Metal is most active is autumn.

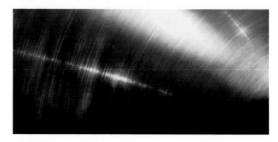

Pathway of the Lung Meridian

Lung is associated with the taking in of breath, transforming it into "true chi" and spreading it throughout the body. Lung is the first line of defence to fight off "external pathogens", which cause diseases such as colds, fevers and flu.

The Lung meridian starts between the first and second ribs, just under the middle of the collarbone, the small bone that links the shoulder to the breastbone. It then travels up crossing the collarbone and across the front of the shoulder, towards the arm. It follows a path down the outside edge of the biceps muscle in the upper arm, through the elbow and towards the wrist. It passes through the wrist, into the hand, and then progresses up the side of the thumb, ending on the outer edge at the corner of the thumbnail.

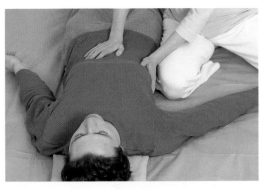

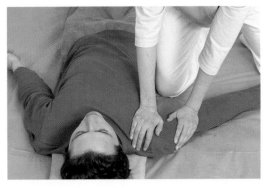

1 Arm straight, palm up Sit in seiza with your hand placed gently on the hara. Bring your partner's arm to an angle of 45 degrees from the body. Lay the arm straight with the palm up.

2 Palm down to the thumb Come into wide leg seiza and move up so that you can stretch towards the shoulders. Palm down Lung meridian all the way down to the thumb.

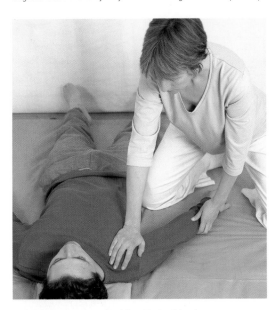

3 Thumb down Lung meridian To do this, change your position so that you are kneeling astride the hand.

Lung meridian points

Two points on Lung meridian are LU 1 and LU 5. Both can be used for respiratory problems, especially for chronic coughs, and prevention of colds and the flu.

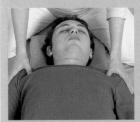

LU 1
Find this point between the first and second ribs, below the middle of the collarbone. This is best accessed from above the head. This is a good point for coughs and chest pain.

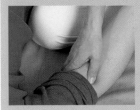

LU 5
This point can be found when you make a fist. It is in the elbow crease at the outside edge of the tendon. LU 5 is good for chronic coughs, arm and elbow pain.

Pathway of the Large Intestine Meridian

The Large Intestine eliminates the waste products of the body. It is like the internal skin, allowing waste products and toxins to pass out of the body. Skin problems, such as acne, and constipation can reflect problems in Large Intestine.

The Large Intestine meridian starts at the corner of the nail of the index finger at the side closest to the thumb. It then travels up the arm, passing through the elbow at the end of the elbow crease on the outside and across the shoulder. It then pursues a course up the side of the neck, crossing the large muscle at the side of the neck towards the nose. The meridian ends at the outside corner of the nostril. Remember that the point LI 4 is contraindicated in pregnancy (see page 47 for more information on contraindications).

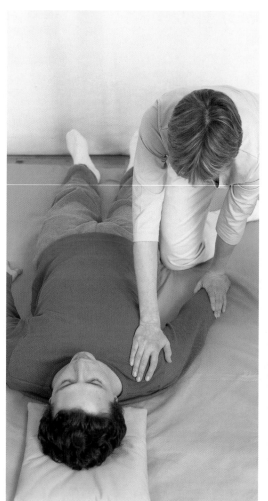

1 Palm up from wrist to elbow Place the arm palm down on the floor alongside the torso. Palm up the meridian from the wrist to the elbow. Move the mother hand to the shoulder. Then use your body weight, coming from the hara, to apply pressure to the shoulder.

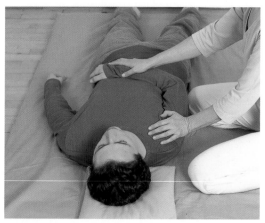

2 Bend arm Bend the arm at right angles and put it across the body so that Large Intestine meridian is at the top of the upper arm. Palm up towards the shoulder.

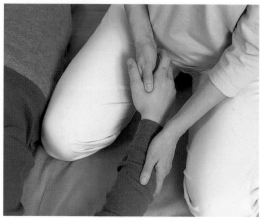

3 Thumb up the meridian To work the meridian with your thumb, bring the arm out to the side and adopt a wide seiza position. Thumb up the meridian – you can hold LI 4 point with your mother hand as you work up the rest of the meridian.

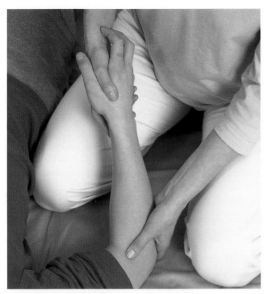

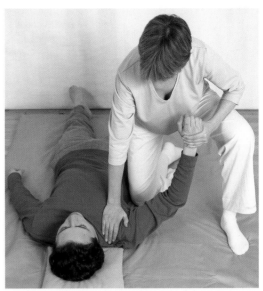

4 Move into point LI 11 Bend the elbow slightly as you go into the point LI 11. This point is on the outside edge of the elbow crease and useful in the prevention of colds, flu, shoulder and arm problems. Hold LI 4 with the other hand.

5 Rotate the arm To make a transition to the other side, lift the arm by the wrist and with mother hand on the shoulder step forward and rotate the arm. Use your mother hand on the shoulder to gauge the ease or stiffness in this joint.

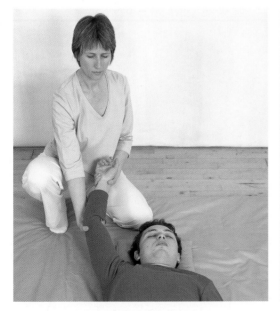

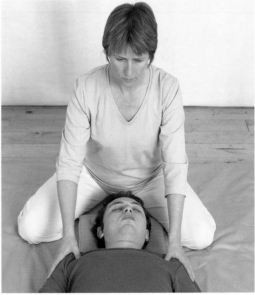

6 Face feet, lean back and stretch arm Step up to the top of the receiver's head, keeping hold of the arm, and turn to face the feet. Lean back and stretch this arm, holding it with one hand under the wrist and the other hand under the elbow.

7 Press into the LU 1 points Reposition yourself in wide seiza above the head and press into the LU 1 points, just below the middle of the collarbones. Move to the other side and work the other arm.

Water

The fluid nature of water means that it can flow into and out of any container, be it a vast ocean or a tiny pool. It is infinitely yielding yet infinitely powerful, ever changing and often dangerous. In nature, without a supply of water, nothing can sprout and grow, flower and blossom and finally be harvested. Water is the ultimate yin: quiet, cold, the resting time of winter. Water's associated meridian pair is Kidney (yin) and Bladder (yang).

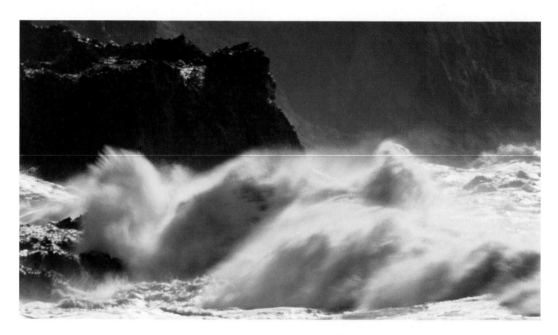

The potential of Water is called the jing or essence. It governs reproduction, fertility and sexual energy. Weakness here can lead to impotence, infertility and reproductive problems. The jing can also be likened to our genes – the constitution we inherit from our ancestors – giving us our vital energy. Water houses the will and give us the impetus to move. The teeth and bones are the related tissue. Weakness in Water can show up as bone disease, lower back pain and sore knees. It controls the water in the body – fluid retention, problems with urination and water metabolism may show imbalance in this element. The sense organ of Water is the ears and hearing.

The emotion associated with water is courage, enabling us to move forward and find new challenges. The converse emotion, fear, is felt if this element is weak. Chronic tiredness can be another symptom of this, as well as a grey complexion, and a dryness in the skin and hair.

Above and below Water can be highly dynamic and powerful, even destructive. It can also have a waiting, silent, still quality that can be described as "stored potential".

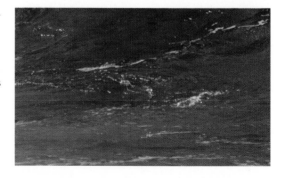

Pathway of the Kidney Meridian

The Kidney stores the jing — our genetic inheritance or constitution. Jing governs
the cycles of life: birth, puberty, reproduction, maturity and death. We are born with
a finite amount of jing and this affects our health, fertility and longevity.

The Kidney meridian starts on the sole of the foot, appearing through the arch on to the inside of the foot. Before it runs up the inside of the leg, there is a small loop, with a number of important points, just above the ankle. The meridian continues up under the main muscles in the front of the thigh and through the groin. It travels up the middle of the front torso, one finger-width either side of the midline until it reaches the ribs, where it branches out (three finger-widths from the midline) and finishes under the inner end of the collarbone.

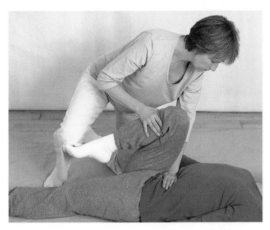

1 Rotate leg With your hand on the hara bring up the leg and rotate, feeling the relative ease or stiffness in the hip joint. Rotate twice to help the joint loosen up.

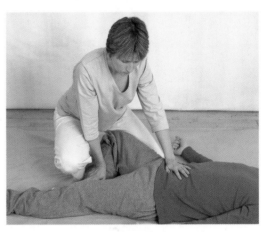

2 Instep against thigh With your hand on the hara let the leg drop out with the instep against the inner thigh of the other leg. Palm up the meridian from the foot to the knee.

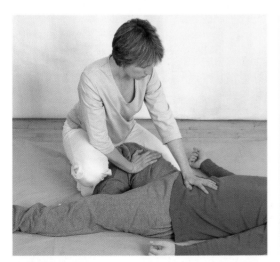

3 Palm up meridian Turn towards your partner's head and continue along the Kidney meridian in the inner thigh, using your mother hand to gauge the depth of pressure.

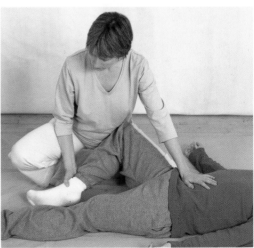

4 Thumb up leg Come back to the ankle and starting at KD 3, thumb up the lower leg. KD 3 is between the inside ankle bone and the Achilles tendon. It helps to strengthen the kidneys.

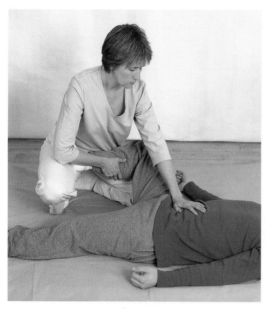

5 Thumb up towards knee Thumb up the meridian towards the knee, and up into the inner thigh, keeping your thumb straight and applying perpendicular pressure.

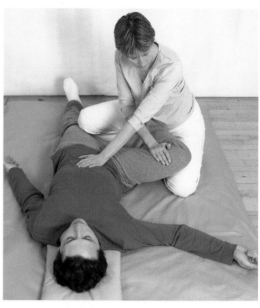

6 Drop leg out You can stretch and open the Kidney meridian by letting the leg drop out so that the knee rests on your thigh. Apply pressure with your palm on the inner thigh.

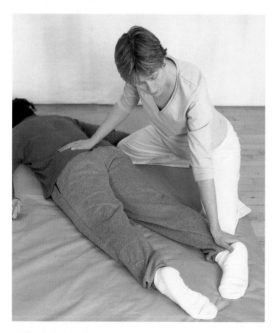

7 Alternative position Lie your partner on their front, turning the feet slightly inwards. Find the point KD 3 on the inside of the ankle between the heel and the ankle bone. Palm up meridian on inside of calf and inside of thigh.

Kidney meridian points

Kidney points can balance the water metabolism and ease problems of the lower back. The first and last points on the Kidney meridian are KD 1 and KD 27. Holding these points will help to stimulate the flow of chi along the whole meridian.

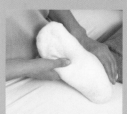

KD 1
This pressure point is on the sole of the foot where the pad of the big toe and the ball of the foot make a "V". This point, known as "Bubbling Spring", is a revitalizing point.

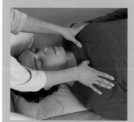

KD 27
This point is nestled in the hollow just below the collarbone at its inner end. This is a good point for coughs and asthma.

Pathway of the Bladder Meridian

Bladder meridian is the longest meridian in the body, starting at the bridge of the nose
and ending at the little toe. Treat Bladder meridian on the back to deeply relax your
partner by calming the central nervous system and balancing all the organ functions.

The Bladder meridian starts either side of the bridge of the
nose, passes over the head and runs down either side of
the spine, dividing at the top of the back into two distinct
lines on each side, that run two finger-widths from the
centre of the spine, and four finger-widths from the centre
of the spine. Between BL13 (between the shoulder blades)
and BL28 (the base of the spine) there are 12 yu points,
which directly influence the 12 organ functions. The
meridian continues down the back of the legs, rejoining
into two single lines at the knee, and ending at the outside
edge of the little toenail. The part of the Bladder meridian
on the back is covered in the basic framework on page 51.

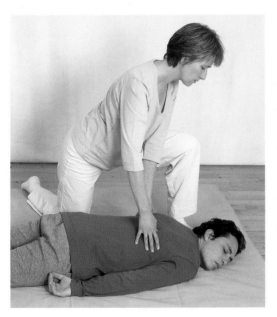

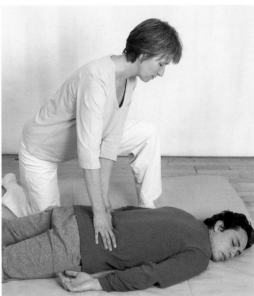

1 Thumb down Thumb down two finger-widths either side
of the mid-line, moving down little by little.

2 BL 23 When you reach the waist, find BL 23, which is in
line with the space between the second and third vertebrae.
This point is good for treating the kidneys and lower back.

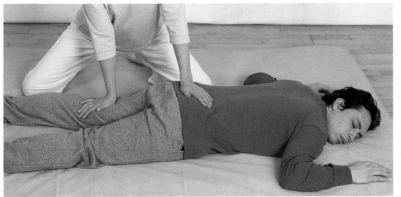

3 Palm down meridian
Repositioning yourself in a
wide seiza position next to
your partner's lower back
and legs, let your mother
hand rest on the sacrum.
Palm down the Bladder
meridian on the leg with
your other hand, using your
body weight to apply
pressure. Avoid pressing
directly on to the back of
the knee.

▷

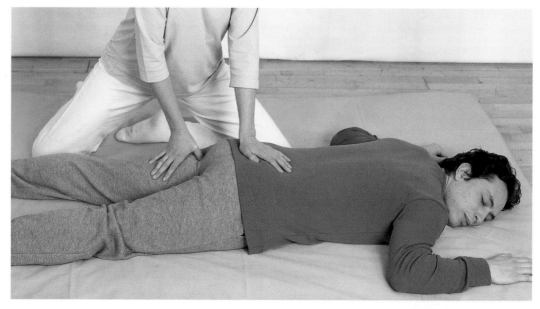

4 Thumb down With the thumb perpendicular to the body, thumb your way down the back of the legs to the knee.

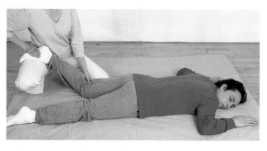

5 Work into the back of the knee Do this by lifting the ankle to bend the knee. BL 40 is in the centre of the crease at the back of the knee – a point good for lower back ache.

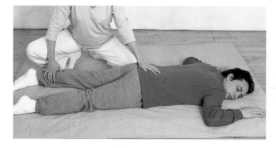

6 Thumb down Continue thumbing down to the ankle. Find BL 57 on the calf muscle halfway between the back of the knee and the heel, another point for lower back ache.

Bladder meridian points

Two important Bladder pressure points on the foot are BL 60 and BL 67. Both points at the opposite end of the meridian from the head, they can be used to treat headaches. They can also be used when working on the foot to improve the flow of chi within the Bladder channel. They can be used with the foot massage as part of the basic framework outline.

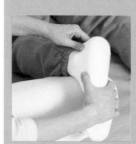

Bladder 60
This point is between the Achilles tendon and the tip of the ankle bone on the outside of the ankle. This is a good point for headache and pain in the neck and occiput. It can also be used for chronic back pain and pain in general.

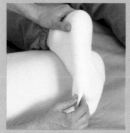

Bladder 67
Locate this point on the outside corner of the base of the little toenail. This can be used for frontal headaches and eye strain. Also used in the last month of pregnancy to turn a breech baby (with caution).

Wood

The energy of the Wood element moves upwards like the growth of a tree. A tree is flexible and can bend in the wind. Flexibility gives us the ability to adapt to circumstances while always growing upwards, towards the light. The function of the Wood element is to make plans and decisions. It harmonizes us and makes all the organs run smoothly. The meridians associated with Wood are the Liver (yin) and Gall Bladder (yang).

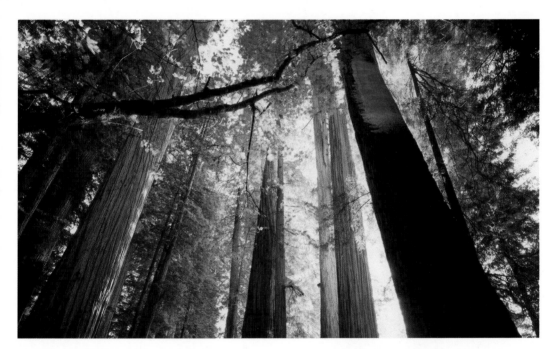

The season for Wood is spring, a time for new growth. If you feel low or hyperactive in spring, you may be suffering from a Wood imbalance. The tissue associated with Wood is the sinews: the nails, tendons and ligaments. Tendons and ligaments cross the joints, holding them together and making smooth, subtle movements possible.

Wood's function is organization and planning. It brings creativity and the intellectual skills required for making things happen. Anger can damage Wood. Repressed anger can lead to a feeling of stuckness and depression. People with Wood problems can be angry and controlling, unable to delegate and prone to workaholism. At the other extreme, they can be stuck, unable to move or make decisions. Look for joint problems, bloating (stuck digestion), headaches (energy stuck in the head), eye problems and brittle nails.

Above and below The function of Wood is organization, planning and creativity, good for bringing a new project to fruition.

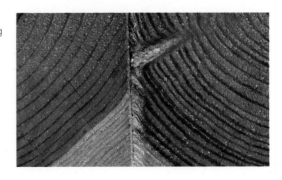

Pathway of the Liver Meridian

Liver governs the smooth flow of chi in the body, ensuring that all the organ
functions are operating in harmony with each other, giving flexibility when needed.
Liver is good for treating headaches, joint problems and premenstrual tension.

The Liver meridian starts at the outside edge of the big toe, at the corner of the toenail. It then passes in front of the ankle bone and pursues a course up the inside of the leg. At the thigh it runs parallel to and above the stringy muscles on the inside of the thigh (the adductors), passing through the groin and continuing up through the belly, across the hara, and finishing under the nipple between the sixth and seventh ribs.

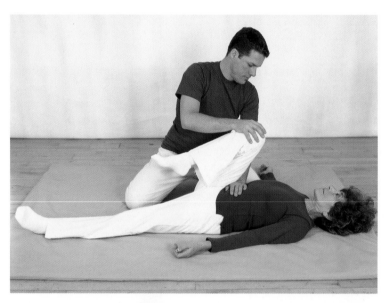

1 Knee up and rotate Sit in a wide seiza position facing your partner, placing your hand on the hara as a mother hand. Pick the leg up from the back of the knee gently and bring the knee up to the body. As you bring the leg up, move your hand to the front of the leg and rotate the leg outwards. Notice any stiffness or restriction as your rotate.

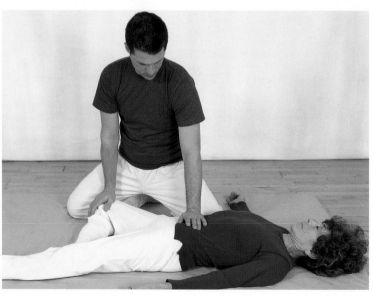

2 Drop knee to side Coming into wide seiza, allow your partner's knee to drop to the side, with the sole of the foot against the inside of the other thigh. If necessary, balance the outstretched knee on your leg for extra support. With your mother hand still on the hara, apply pressure gently downwards to open up Liver meridian and to stretch the thigh. Ask your partner to let you know if they feel any pain or discomfort.

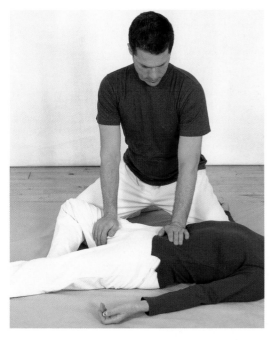

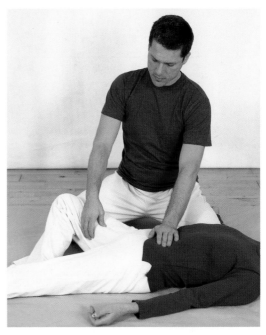

3 Palm up Move up the meridian, up the lower leg and inner thigh, keeping your mother hand on the hara.

4 Thumb up slowly Thumb your way up the meridian taking care to go in slowly and with perpendicular pressure.

Liver meridian points

Four main landmark points on the Liver meridian are LV 3, LV 8, LV 13 and LV 14. LV 3, LV 13 and LV 14 are very good general points for unblocking Liver chi stagnation. Symptoms of stagnation include bloating, digestive problems, depression, moodiness, premenstrual tension and irregular periods. As well as moving stagnation, each of these points will have a specific action.

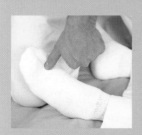

LV 3
This point is two finger-widths below the webbing between the big toe and the second toe. An important point and often painful, it is used for migraine headaches and can be used for calming frustration.

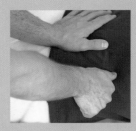

LV 13
This point is at the free end of the eleventh floating rib. It is a good point for treating digestive problems that result in diarrhoea.

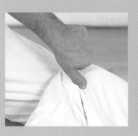

LV 8
Locate this point by bending the knee and it is at the end of the knee crease on the inside leg. Very often painful, this is a useful point for knee problems.

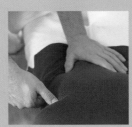

LV 14
Find this point between the sixth and seventh ribs directly below the nipple. Good for treating digestive problems that result in nausea and vomiting.

Pathway of the Gall Bladder Meridian

Gall Bladder is important in the process of decision-making and can become out of balance in people with high-level jobs. Its position on the head, neck and shoulders makes it ideal for treating headaches and shoulder tension caused by stress.

The Gall Bladder meridian starts at the outside corner of the eye and circles around the back of the ear and the side of the head, making three concentric arcs. It runs down the back of the neck, crosses the shoulder and runs in front of the ball and socket joint of the shoulder to the side of the body under the armpit. It then zigzags towards the front ribs and back to the hip, continuing down the side of the leg and ending at the outside edge of the fourth toe at the nail. Remember that the point GB 21 is contraindicated during pregnancy.

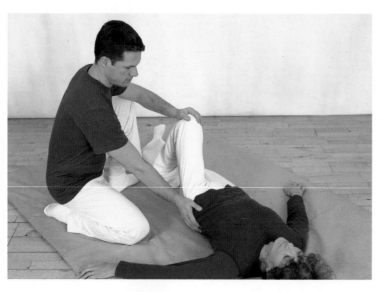

1 Lift leg from under knee
Sit with one knee up and one down and bring the leg into position to treat Gall Bladder by lifting the leg from under the knee. Bend up the leg and place your partner's foot next to the other knee. Bring your hand on to the front of the knee to support it as your mother hand rests on the hip.

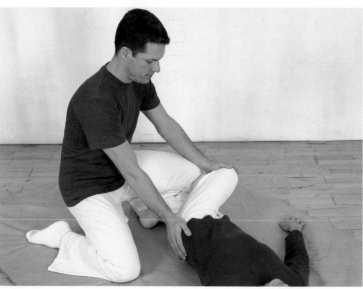

2 Stretch the meridian Adjust your hand so that the palm is on the outside of the knee, forming a base from which pressure can be applied. Gently push the leg down towards the floor over the other leg, which remains on the floor. Keep your mother hand on the hip throughout, applying pressure to prevent the hip from rising off the floor. Ask your partner to tell you if you are over stretching or causing discomfort.

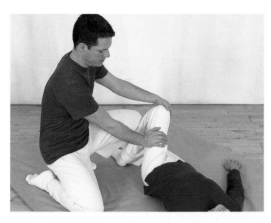

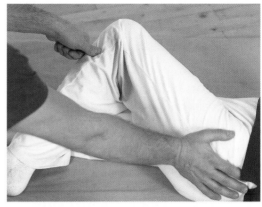

3 Support the calf with your knee and put your foot against your partner's foot to anchor it. Palm down the meridian.

4 Thumb down the meridian with the mother hand on the hip, moving it on to the knee as you move down the leg.

Gall Bladder meridian points

As it travels through most of the major joints, the Gall Bladder meridian is good for joint problems, particularly the knee and hip joints. There are seven important landmark points on the Gall Bladder meridian: GB 1 and GB 44 (the first and last points) and GB 20, GB 21, GB 31, GB 34 and GB 40.

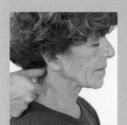

GB 20
This point is under the base of the skull, halfway between the mid-line and the lower edge of the skull. Press the thumb up towards the forehead for the correct angle. Good for neck tension and headaches.

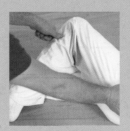

GB 34
This point is in a hollow under and in front of the small head of the fibula below the knee (the bone on the outside of the leg). A general point for joint problems and for treating the knee.

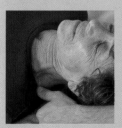

GB 21
This point is located mid-way along the shoulder on the highest point. It is nearly always painful and is good for a stiff, painful or frozen shoulder. Not to be used during pregnancy.

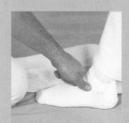

GB 40
In the hollow in front of and underneath the external ankle bone. This point can be used to treat ankle problems and is good for freeing stuck Liver energy and for helping decision-making.

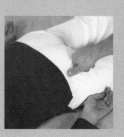

GB 31
Find this point one-third of the distance between the hip and the bottom of the sacrum in the hollow. This is a useful point for treating hip problems and sciatica.

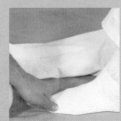

GB 44
Located at the outside edge of the fourth toe just at the corner of the toenail. Effective for headaches around the eyes as well as for red, sore eyes.

Primary Fire

The Fire element embodies consciousness or spirit, the spark of life. Fire gives warmth and is active. While it can blaze with energy, it can also be calming: through the beat of the heart Fire creates a constant and stable rhythm in the body. It governs the emotions and how we interpret our environment through them. The blood vessels and the circulation are controlled by Primary Fire, and the associated meridian pair is Heart (yin) and Small Intestine (yang).

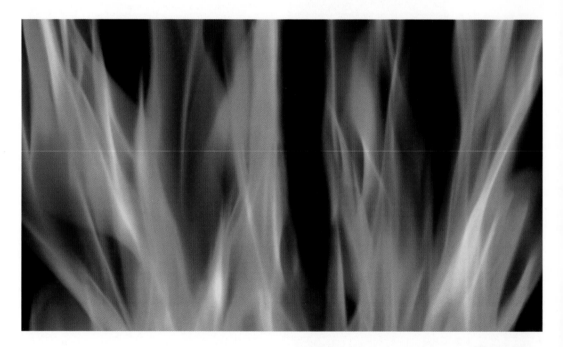

The emotions related to Fire are love and joy. Long-term stress can damage the heart and create hysteria. The emotions can become chaotic and erratic. A person with strong Fire energy may laugh a lot – and is likely to be a comedian. The functions of Fire are communication and awareness, and the Fire inside us will let us know how we are affected by the external world. Conditions caused by Fire imbalances include heart disease, poor circulation and difficulty in assimilating nutrients through the small intestine. The season associated with Fire is the summer, and if you feel hot and bothered at this time of year, it may indicate that you have too much Fire energy. The taste is bitter. The colour of Fire is red – someone with a red face may be showing an imbalance in Fire.

Above and below Fire provides the emotions of love and joy, although too much Fire can lead to over-excitement or hysteria.

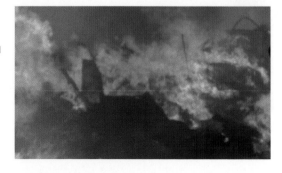

Pathway of the Heart Meridian

The Heart houses the shen which can be translated as "spirit" or "consciousness".
The shen must be rooted and stable and needs a calm heart. Imbalances in shen
can show up as insomnia, disturbing dreams and, in extreme cases, mental illness.

The Heart meridian starts under the armpit, within the hollow that forms when you hold your arm right up. With the arm by the side and the palm towards the front it travels down the inside of the arm, along the inside edge of the biceps muscle. It passes through the elbow and along the inside of the wrist towards the palm. Passing along the little finger side, it ends at the little finger on the side nearest the ring finger at the base of the nail.

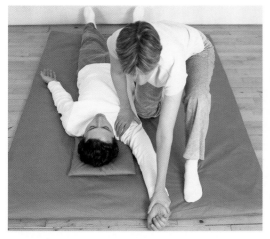

1 Open up the Heart meridian Hold the arm loosely by the wrist and step forward, lifting the arm vertical and then bringing it up over the head, pushing to stretch the arm.

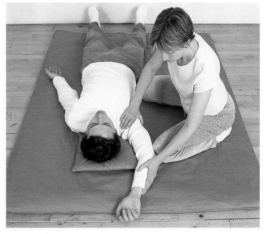

2 Place the arm in position for Heart meridian Release the wrist and bend the arm slightly, allowing it to lie comfortably above the head.

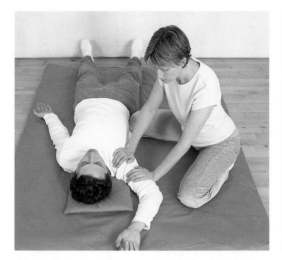

3 Palm up Work up the meridian from the armpit on the outside of the arm towards the little finger. Keep your mother hand on the shoulder.

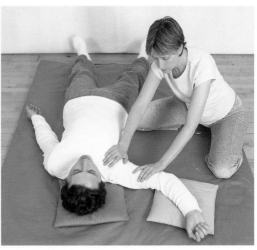

4 Variation If your partner's arm is uncomfortable pointing straight up you can put the arm slightly more out to the side and rest it on a cushion.

▷

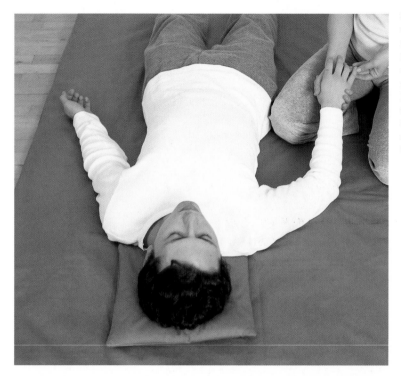

5 Working the hand When working the points in the hand (see HT 7 and HT 9 below) sit back in seiza by your partner's side and bring the arm down to rest it on your thigh. Turn the hand palm side up to work along the edge of the palm and turn it palm side down to work on the little finger – the end of the meridian.

Heart meridian points

There are four landmark points on the Heart meridian: HT 1, HT 3, HT 7 and HT 9. The two hand points can be treated when working on the hands. Caution should be taken when treating someone with a serious cardiovascular condition and beginners should avoid this altogether. If in doubt refer them to a more experienced practitioner.

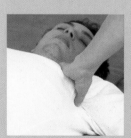

HT 1
This point is located in the deepest part of the armpit at the centre. It can be used for treating insomnia.

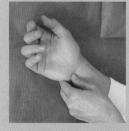

HT 7
Located in the crease on the side of the wrist nearest the little finger, this point calms anxiety and worry caused by stress, and helps with insomnia.

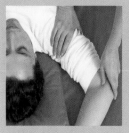

HT 3
This point is located at the end of the elbow crease at the little finger side of the arm. It calms the mind and can be used for elbow problems.

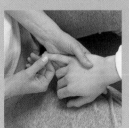

HT 9
This point is at the end of the little finger at the inside corner of the fingernail. This is a revival point in cases of heart attack.

Pathway of the Small Intestine Meridian

The function of the small intestine is to assimilate nourishment. It receives food
from the spleen and separates the pure from the impure. The pure is assimilated
and the impure is sent to the large intestine for elimination.

The Small Intestine meridian starts at the outside edge
of the little finger, runs along the back of the arm and
passes through the space between the ulna and the
humerus on the little finger side. It then travels along
the back of the arm towards the back of the shoulder.
After this, it does a zigzag on the scapula and moves up
the neck behind the big muscle at the side of the neck,
ending just in front of the ear.

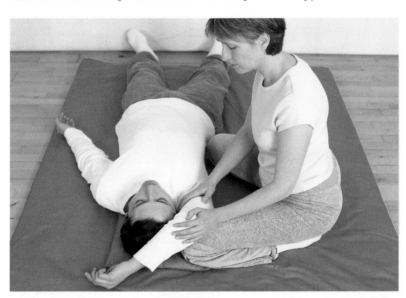

**1 Expose Small Intestine
meridian** Bring your
partner's arm up over the
head so that the elbow is
pointing up and the side of
the arm is uppermost. This
position will expose the
Small Intestine meridian.
You can support the arm
on your thigh so that it can
relax. Hold the upper arm
with your hand.

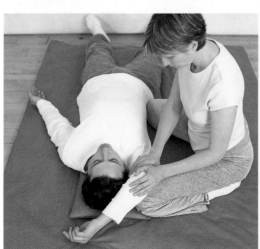

2 Work from wrist to armpit Palm down the Small Intestine
meridian from wrist to armpit. Have your mother hand on the
elbow when working from the elbow towards the shoulder.

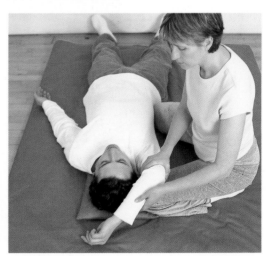

3 Thumb down Work down the meridian from the wrist
towards the elbow. When you reach the elbow, change your
mother hand to the elbow and continue towards the shoulder. ▷

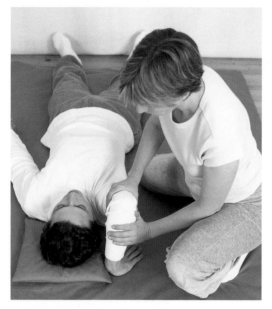

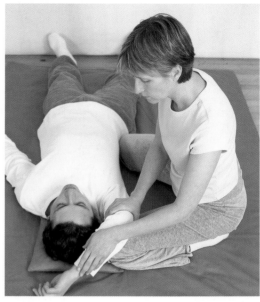

4 Variation This alternative position for working the Small Intestine meridian involves pointing the elbow up and placing the palm of the hand on the ground next to the head with the fingers pointing towards the shoulder.

4b Variation Palm the meridian from wrist to shoulder. This is a good position for opening up the Small Intestine meridian but is better used on people who are more flexible in the shoulder.

Small Intestine meridian points

The Small Intestine meridian is important for treating shoulder problems as the meridian crosses the shoulder blade. Shock is also very often treated by working Small Intestine meridian (the body's inability to assimilate). Four important landmark points on the Small Intestine meridian are SI 1, SI 8, SI 11 and SI 19.

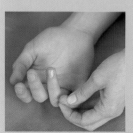

SI 1
This point is found on the end of the little finger at the outside corner of the fingernail. It is good for treating a stiff neck.

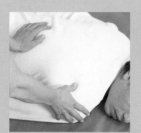

SI 11
Located in the middle of the shoulder blade in the depression, this point is always a painful point and very good for shoulder pain.

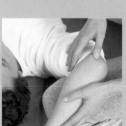

SI 8
This point is located at the back of the elbow in the hollow between the two bones on the little finger side. It can be used for elbow and neck pain and helps to calm the mind.

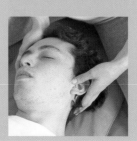

SI 19
This point is found in the hollow in front of the middle of the ear formed when opening the mouth. Use it to treat deafness and tinnitus.

Secondary Fire

Secondary Fire shares the same characteristics as Primary Fire. The meridians associated with Secondary Fire are Heart Protector (yin) and Triple Heater (yang), functions with no Western equivalent but which could be described as Circulation and Protection. Heart Protector protects the heart, and Triple Heater governs the peripheral circulation. Together they are responsible for a healthy and balanced emotional state.

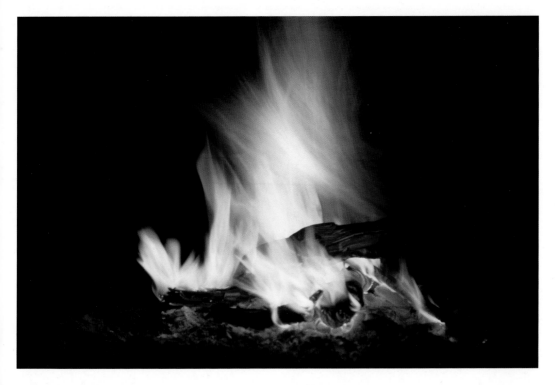

The Heart Protector acts as a buffer for the heart and protects it from physical and emotional trauma. The Heart Protector is often seen as the relationship meridian – emotional trauma will deeply affect the Heart Protector. When relationships go wrong, we can become very protective of our heart, bringing energy into the Heart Protector. It also governs the circulation, and conditions such as varicose veins and high blood pressure can show up as an imbalance in this function.

The Triple Heater governs what are known as the "three burning spaces" in the body: the upper, middle and lower burners. The Triple Heater keeps them in

Above The Triple Heater keeps the "three burning spaces" in balance and acts as the body's thermostat.

balance. Each space corresponds to certain internal organs: the upper heater is the heart and lungs, the middle heater is the stomach and spleen and the lower heater is the kidney, bladder, liver, and small and large intestines.

Symptoms associated with the Triple Heater function can be feeling the cold and difficulty in adapting to the environment. Those suffering from low Triple Heater energy may have a low immune system function, and it can also lead to other auto-immune problems such as allergies.

Pathway of the Heart Protector Meridian

Heart Protector supports the heart, protecting it from both physical and emotional pressure. It is associated with the pericardium, the outer layer of tissue which surrounds the heart. It can help open the chest and ease emotional problems.

The Heart Protector meridian starts at the side of the breast, adjacent to the armpit. It runs up above the armpit and then travels down the centre of the inside of the arm, passing through the elbow and wrist between the Heart and Lung meridians. It ends on the front of the middle finger, at the very tip.

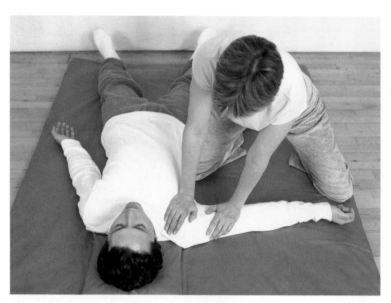

1 Palming Start in seiza position next to your partner. Turn your body slightly towards the head and pick up the arm lightly by the wrist. Lift and place it back on the floor so that it is at right angles to the body. Keep the palm facing upwards, and place your mother hand gently on the shoulder. Use your other hand to palm all the way down the Heart Protector meridian, from the shoulder down the middle of the arm to the middle finger.

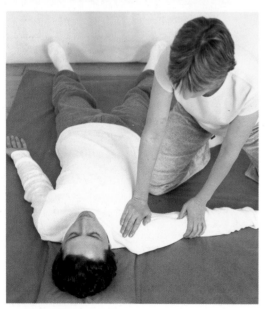

2 Thumb down to elbow Keep your mother hand on the shoulder, and thumb the Heart Protector meridian from the shoulder to the elbow.

Heart Protector

The function of the Heart Protector does not have an equivalent in Western medicine, the nearest being the pericardium, the protective tissue which surrounds the heart. In Chinese medicine the Heart was described as the Emperor or supreme controller overseeing the spiritual health of his subjects. The Heart Protector was the ambassador who guarded the functions of the supreme controller and shielded the spirit from danger, so that internal peace and harmony was restored.

In some early texts the Heart was seen as sacred and so was rarely treated. Heart can be treated through the Heart Protector meridian, especially in cases of emotional trauma. Heart Protector particularly governs the circulation of the body and can be used effectively to treat mild cases of high blood pressure.

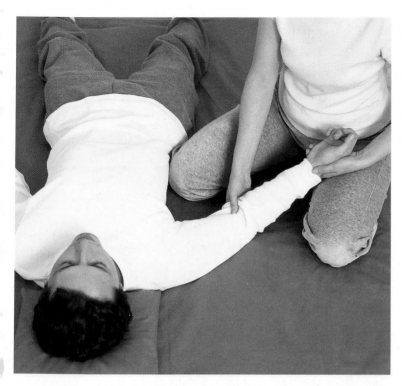

3 Thumb down from elbow to finger When you reach the elbow, bend it slightly as you go in with your thumb. This will allow you to go in deeper. Continue down the lower arm until you reach the hand, finishing at the tip of the middle finger. Ask your partner to keep the arm relaxed.

Heart Protector meridian points

You can treat the Heart Protector meridian in cases of some cardiovascular conditions, such as high blood pressure and mild angina, rather than working directly on Heart meridian. Four main landmark points on Heart Protector meridian are HP 3, HP 6, HP 8 and HP 9. All these, except for HP 9, will help to release anxiety.

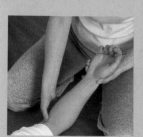

HP 3
This point is located on the elbow crease on the inside of the tendon you feel when bending the arm. This point can be used to calm the mind in cases of anxiety and to treat nausea and vomiting.

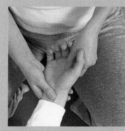

HP 8
Find this point in the centre of the palm – fold the fingers down and it is where the middle finger touches the palm. This point calms the mind and is good for exam nerves.

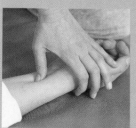

HP 6
This point is located three finger-widths below the wrist crease in between the two tendons. A very useful point for nausea and travel sickness. Calms the mind and relieves chest pain.

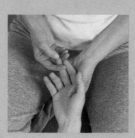

HP 9
This point is at the tip of the middle finger. It is the last point on the meridian and is a revival point.

Pathway of the Triple Heater Meridian

Triple Heater governs the "three burning spaces" roughly equivalent to the chest cavity, the solar plexus area and the lower abdomen. It ensures that these areas maintain their correct temperatures and that the organs are working harmoniously.

The Triple Heater meridian starts at the fourth, or ring, finger at the base of the nail on the outside edge, nearest to the little finger. It then runs along the back of the arm and passes through the elbow joint on the thumb side of the arm. It then travels along the back of the shoulder, up the back of the neck, behind and around the ear and finishes at the very outside corner of the eyebrow.

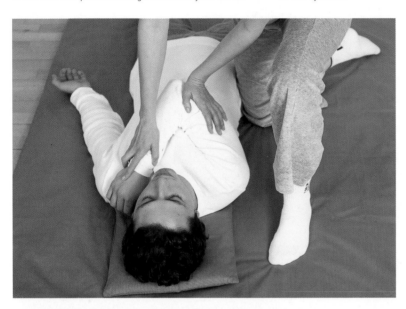

1 Stretch arm Bring the arm across the body so that Triple Heater meridian will be exposed on the top of the arm. With one hand just above the elbow and the other hand on the wrist you can stretch the arm towards the opposite shoulder to open up the back of the shoulder and open up Triple Heater on the upper arm. Check with your partner – sometimes women can find this stretch uncomfortable.

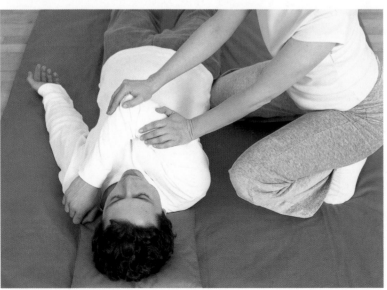

2 Palm up Placing your top hand down on to the elbow to become the mother hand, palm your way up from the wrist to the elbow and then, changing hands, from the elbow to the shoulder. Make sure that your pressure is perpendicular to the arm and not pushing the arm on to the chest, which can be uncomfortable and constrict the breathing.

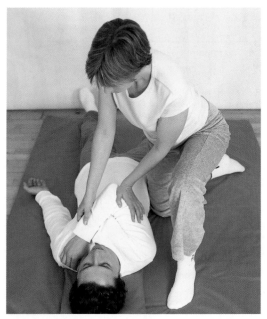

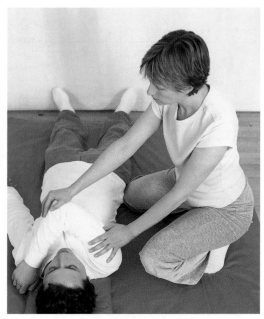

3 Thumb down Returning your mother hand to the upper arm, just above the elbow, thumb down the forearm. Once again make sure that your partner can breathe freely.

4 Thumb upper arm Swap your mother hand, so that your mother hand now rests on the elbow. You can now thumb the upper arm with the other hand.

Triple Heater meridian points
The main landmark points on Triple Heater meridian are TH 4, TH 10, TH 15 and TH 23. Triple Heater is like the thermostat of the body, so fevers or excessive cold will affect its functioning. It governs peripheral circulation, and cold hands or feet reflect a problem in Triple Heater.

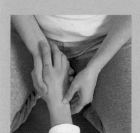

TH 4
This point is located in the back of the wrist joint in a depression in line with the fourth finger. This point is good for headaches and shoulder pain.

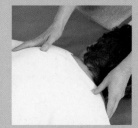

TH 15
This point is one thumb width below GB 21 (see page 89). Use it for shoulder and neck pain and stiffness.

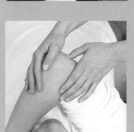

TH 10
Bend the elbow and this point is in the depression one thumb-width above the point of the elbow. This point is good for tennis elbow, elbow pain and stiffness in general.

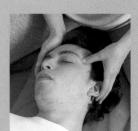

TH 23
This point is in the hollow at the outside tip of the eyebrow. It is good for eye problems and headaches.

The Conception Vessel

Considered as an "extraordinary" meridian, the Conception Vessel is not usually
treated like the other meridians. There are important points on this meridian, called
Bo points, which can be used to treat and diagnose the energy of other meridians.

The Conception Vessel, running down the centre of the body, governs all the yin channels and is a reservoir of energy for these channels. It influences all stages of conception and pregnancy and the female reproductive system. It can be used to strengthen the yin energy of the body. There are points called Bo points on the Conception Vessel which relate to individual meridians

and these points can be used to treat and diagnose their corresponding meridian, especially its emotional and spiritual aspects. The Conception Vessel starts at CV1, a point on the perineum between the anus and the genital organs. It continues up through the front of the body on the mid-line and ends just under the lower lip. CV 1 and CV 8 in the umbilicus are contraindicated points.

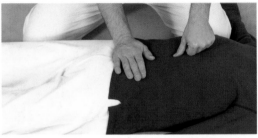

2 Hold CV 12, located midway between the navel and the lower end of the sternum, good for stomach problems.

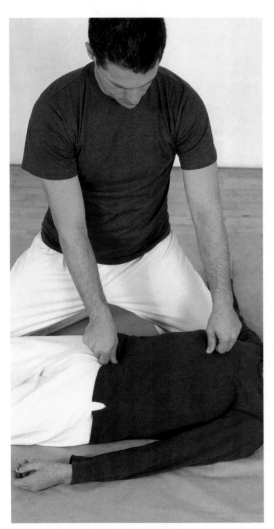

1 Hold the points CV 6 and CV 17 and feel the energy between these points, connecting the Heart and the hara.

Conception Vessel points
All the yin channels are governed by the Conception Vessel, which acts like a reservoir of energy for these pathways. CV 6 and CV 17, mentioned earlier, are important points on the Conception Vessel meridian, linking the whole system.

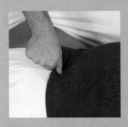

CV 6
This point is two finger-widths below the navel. It is known as "Sea of chi", and is an important point because it builds up chi. It can be used for physical and mental exhaustion and depression.

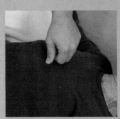

CV 17
Located in between the nipples on the mid-line, this point is important in relation to the Heart Protector (called a Bo point) and has a beneficial effect on the chest, easing pain and tightness in the chest.

The Governing Vessel

Running along the spine, the Governing Vessel plays a similar role to the
Conception Vessel, for the yang meridians instead of the yin. It can be used for
strengthening the spine and nervous system.

The Governing Vessel governs all the yang meridians.
It is a reservoir of energy for these meridians and can
be used to strengthen all the yang energy in the body.
It influences the spine, the brain and the kidney.

Imbalances in the Governing Vessel will affect the
spine and the nervous system on a deep level.
Conditions such as epilepsy and serious spinal

degeneration may result. Governing Vessel can have a
beneficial effect on the spirit and mind. GV 20 is an
especially good point for lifting the spirits.

The Governing Vessel starts at a point between the
anus and the base of the coccyx. It follows the mid-line
of the spine, continuing over the head, and finishes at a
point under the top lip on the gum.

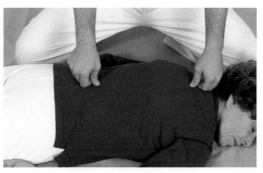

2 Find and hold GV 4, which is between the second and
third lumbar vertebrae. This is an important point for
stimulating Kidney energy and for easing any lower
back problems.

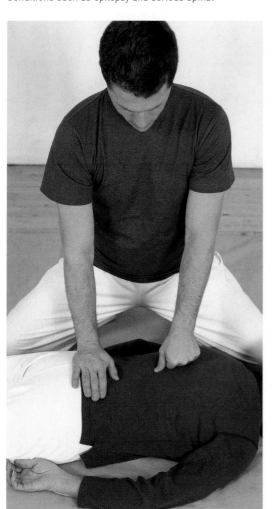

1 You can work on Governing Vessel meridian by finding
individual points down the spine. Notice where there is a
kyo area in the back and hold there.

Governing Vessel points
Two other points of interest on the Governing Vessel
are GV 16 and GV 20.

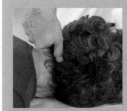

GV 16
Find this point in the
hollow on the mid-line
just below the base of
the skull. This point
clears the mind and
stimulates the brain.

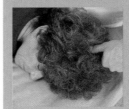

GV 20
Located on an imaginary
line between the tips of
the ears, and on the
mid-line, this point has
a strong lifting action. It
can lift depression and is
used for haemorrhoids.

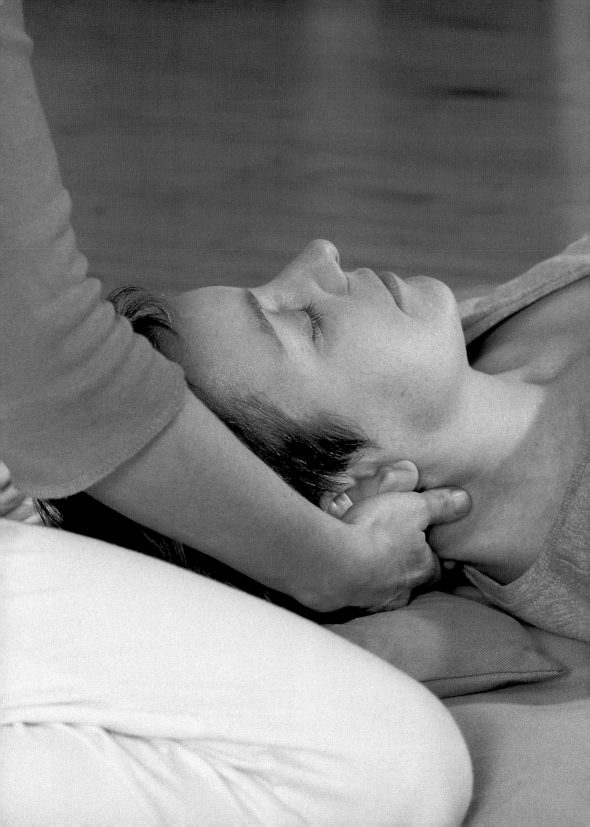

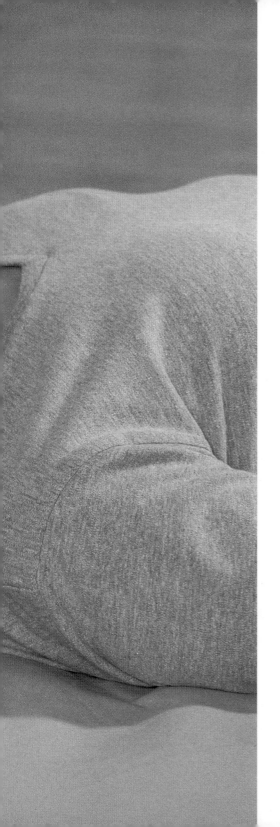

A Full
Treatment

Usually a treatment takes an hour from start to finish, with the actual hands-on part lasting about 35–40 minutes. This gives you time to take a case history and make a diagnosis at the beginning, perform the full treatment, and have some time left at the end for your partner to recover and for you to advise them on further action to take.

In this section we look at how to put everything together. The first part is the art of diagnosis – how to assess your partner so that you can devise the best possible treatment to address his or her particular condition. There are four methods of diagnosis: looking, listening and smelling, questioning, and touching. After that we follow a full treatment, showing how to put a session together and decide on any recommendations.

Diagnosis

Evaluation and advice play a central role in Shiatsu. The first stage is to gather information about the receiver so that an assessment can be made in relation to any energy or elemental imbalances. A treatment appropriate to the condition can then be decided upon. Shiatsu diagnosis is not a medical evaluation and, if you suspect that your partner has a medical condition, you should advise him or her to seek medical advice.

To develop good diagnostic skills in Shiatsu you have to observe carefully and develop your intuition. Intuition is really just a finely developed form of observation.

In traditional Eastern medicine there are four methods used to assess a client's condition: looking, listening and smelling, questioning, and touching.

LOOKING
This includes observing areas such as style of dress, hygiene, presentation, skin tone, posture and energy patterns. Immediately your partner comes into sight you will unconsciously begin to assess his or her condition. Is your partner fidgety, upright and tense, or lazy, hunched and slow to react?

Influenced by our cultural and social conditioning we will make judgements based on gender, age, appearance, style of dress, and so on. Many people present themselves to reflect their inner countenance, by dressing in bright colours, for example. We naturally make intuitive assessments of our partner's health based on our observation. We may say "you're looking well" or "you look a bit off colour". In Shiatsu we seek to formalize these assessments by looking for particular markers, such as face colour, hair, posture, and so on.

KYO AND JITSU
These terms are both used to describe the presence or absence of chi in the meridians and in areas of the body. An overall impression can be gained about the relative kyo or jitsu condition of a person: do they appear to be full of energy or do they look weak and tired?

In a more kyo condition, the person is slumped, the belly is sagging or the shoulders are rounded. There is a lack of vitality, tiredness and shallow breathing. Kyo people can be thin and frail or obese and sluggish.

In a more jitsu condition, a person has a high level of tension. They can have hyperactive, jerky movements and a more stiff posture, possibly with chest thrust out and the shoulders held back.

Below and below opposite Look at your partner's posture from all sides, standing and walking. Look for energy imbalances.

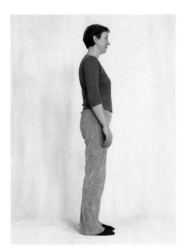
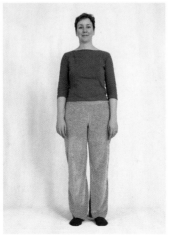
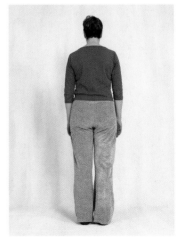

POSTURE

Bad postural habits develop over many years and can be a response to an internal condition, an emotional problem or some kind of trauma. We tend to want to protect weakness and veer away from pain. For example, if someone has a painful ankle they usually put more weight on the other foot to protect the bad ankle and walk with a limp. After a while this can become a habitual way of walking and, even when the pain has receded, the habit may remain. The body may adapt to this change and, as the body compensates, this could result in other postural habits developing.

Looking at the posture will give you clues as to areas of weakness, pain and tension in the body and the emotional state of your partner. Observe the posture from the front, the back and sides, and walking if you can. Take note of the following questions:

- What do you notice first?
- Is one shoulder higher than the other?
- Is one arm longer than the other?
- Are the shoulders rounded or tense?
- When walking is there a part of the body that doesn't move, such as the shoulders or hips?
- Does one arm move more than the other?
- Is there a trace of a limp?
- Is the head thrust forward, or leaning?
- Is the body stooping or hunched?

If you see any of the above conditions, for example rounded shoulders, this can be an area you can address in your treatment. Look at your partner's posture again after the treatment and see if it has changed. In your recommendations, you may want to suggest that your partner improves their posture, giving pointers to the areas to be addressed.

Posture exercise

Get together with a partner and watch them walking towards and away from you

- See if you can copy their walk
- How does it feel to walk like them?
- Can you sense an imbalance?
- Can you locate an area that needs attention?
- Are there areas of tension you notice or feelings you have walking in this way?
- Does your partner recognize the posture when you copy them, and notice the postural habits?
- Can you make any suggestions to improve this posture?

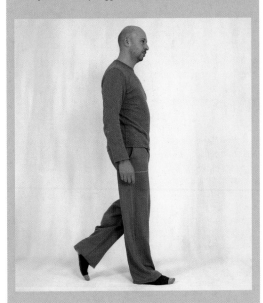

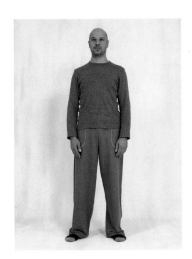

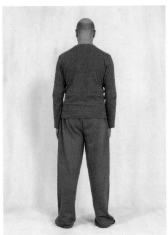

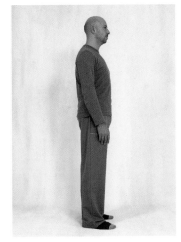

Facial Diagnosis

The face is a reflection of a person's health. The condition of the skin and the vitality in the eyes show the energy levels of the five elements, and the colour or hue of the face shows the element that is out of balance. Each part of the face is related to a specific body organ, set of functions and element. A fullness or an emptiness in any of these areas demonstrates that there is an imbalance within that meridian.

The face can be divided into different areas, each relating to one of the organ functions. Skin blemishes or discoloration in one of these areas may show some imbalance or build-up of toxins in that organ. For example the tip of the nose represents Heart and under the eyes represents Kidney. A redness in the end of the nose can indicate circulation problems, and dark bags under the eyes may show that Kidney is under stress.

In Shiatsu, a person's constitution – their reproductive health, longevity and resistance to disease – tends to show up in the face. Strong, prominent eyebrows show power and vitality, especially in Liver, Kidney and Triple Heater. A healthy head of hair is believed to indicate good sexual energy, again relating to the Kidney energy.

The size of the ears is linked to the health of Kidney, a meridian that governs vital essence, reproductive health and longevity. A good exercise to gauge the strength of the ears is to take firm hold of both ears and gently pull and rotate them to see how rooted they are. If they move easily then Kidney (and the constitution) may be weak. Large earlobes, as well as being considered a sign of longevity, are thought to indicate wisdom.

Look also for colour or hue of the face, which will often show the element that is out of balance. For example, someone who is red-faced may have problems in the Fire element and this could indicate cardiovascular problems, such as high blood pressure. A very pale-faced person may have Lung problems.

The shape of the face

In Shiatsu, you should also look at the shape and structure of the face. If the shape of the face is rectangular or oval with high cheekbones and pale hair, the person is likely to have more of a Metal personality and could be creative or intuitive. A longer face that is more triangular indicates a Wood person who tends to be decisive and goal-oriented. A square-shaped face, with a square jaw and broad features, is probably an Earth personality – someone who is practical, stable and grounded. A Fire personality is likely to have a more pointed face and chin, maybe with red hair and freckles or a redder complexion, and therefore likely to be be enthusiastic and inspirational. A rounder, softer face, usually with dark hair, may be a Water personality who will be sociable, wise and more in touch with their emotions.

Many people will have a mixture of the five elements in the shape of the face, and there will not always be one prominent element.

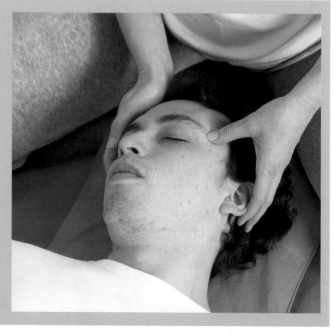

The Face Map

A person's constitution – including reproductive health, longevity and resistance to disease – will show up in the face. For example, redness on the end of the nose or upper cheeks can indicate cardiovascular problems relating to Heart.

This diagram shows the different areas of the face and how they relate to each element and the organs of the body. The face can be divided into different areas, each relating to one of the organ functions. Look at the diagram of the face: the colours show the areas of the face that are represented by each element. Look for skin blemishes, discoloration (particularly one of the colours relating to one of the five elements), puffiness or lines in any of these areas. This will show some imbalance or build-up of energy or toxins in that organ and element.

For example, dark patches under the eyes show conditions in Stomach, Liver and Kidney. If they are bluish, Kidney may be under stress; if the discoloration is more greenish, it could indicate a build-up of toxins in the liver. Redness on the end of the nose or on the upper cheeks shows cardiovascular problems relating to Heart. Pallid, white or sunken cheeks can indicate a Lung weakness. A swollen lower lip could show a sluggish or weak large intestine. Prominence of the V-shaped forehead wrinkles indicates Gall Bladder conditions.

Gall Bladder
Look for excessive lines or discoloration, maybe greenish, in this area on the forehead. Above the eyebrows you may see small V-shaped wrinkles.

Kidney
Under the eyes, dark blue circles show stress in Kidney, or bluish puffiness may show water retention. Puffiness or discoloration on the chin can be kidney related.

Lung
The lower cheeks will reflect a Lung condition. Look for grey or pallid cheeks, sometimes pitted, spotty or sunken.

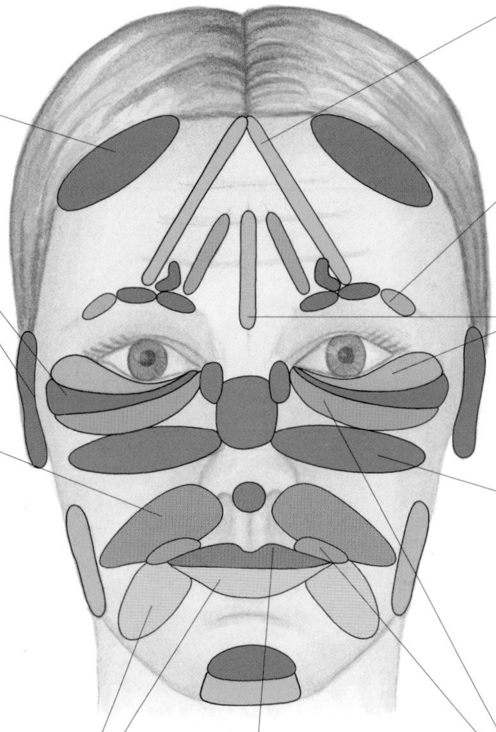

Key to the meridians

- Gall Bladder
- Large and Small Intestine
- Stomach
- Triple Heater
- Heart
- Bladder
- Spleen
- Liver
- Lung
- Kidney

Bladder
Two strong lines on the forehead will indicate some stress in Bladder. Sometimes you will see puffiness, pitting or discoloration on the lower chin.

Triple Heater
Very little hair at the end of the eyebrows or the eyebrows being short can indicate an imbalance in Triple Heater.

Stomach
A deep central line between the eyebrows, a yellowish colour directly under the eyes or yellowish, sunken or pitted skin at the side of cheeks indicate problems.

Heart
Look for redness or broken veins along the bridge of the nose and top of cheeks. The tip of the nose may additionally be red and swollen. (Heart Protector doesn't have a specific area of the face, but will be the same as Heart and sometimes shows up as a red complexion.)

Large and Small Intestine
A swollen lower lip or blemishes here indicate problems in the small or large intestines. For Large Intestine you may also see deep lines at the side of the mouth.

Spleen
The area above the mouth indicates Spleen conditions. Look for a yellowish discoloration, puffiness or blemishes.

Liver
A greenish puffiness at the upper corner of the mouth or under the eyes shows stagnation in the Liver. Two deep frown lines between the eyebrows can indicate excess anger affecting Liver.

Listening and Smelling

The sound of the voice and a person's body odour give you a clue to the element that is out of balance. Look at the table below to see the correspondences of voice and smell with each element. Diagnosis by listening means assessing the sound and tone of the voice to see if it has a particular characteristic. Body smell can be related to different organs within the five element system, as shown in the correspondences table.

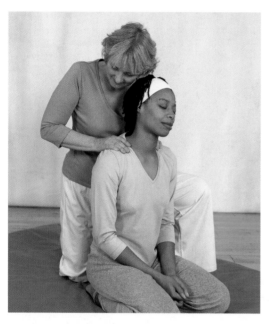

SENSITIVE EVALUATION

Listening is not just hearing what your partner has to say, but also the way in which it is said. A listening assessment can begin during the first phone call or initial contact by noting the tone of voice. Sometimes it helps to listen with your eyes closed and hear it as if you were listening to music. You are looking for a predominance of a tone of voice which may not necessarily be in harmony with what they are saying. A weeping, weak or breathy voice relates to the Metal element. A laughing, hearty voice can indicate a Fire personality, and those who laugh for no reason may have a Fire imbalance. Those with an Earth personality will exhibit a sing-song or lilting voice.

The smell is more difficult to assess in Shiatsu as the receiver remains clothed, although in some cases you may be able to pick up a distinctive odour. Acupuncturists smell the area just below the back of the neck by lifting the back of the collar. This area is less likely to be washed regularly as it is difficult to reach.

Left Listening and smelling can be performed while in the process of massaging the neck and shoulders – this will put your partner at their ease.

Five Element organs, seasons and senses

	WOOD	**FIRE**	**EARTH**	**METAL**	**WATER**
YIN ORGAN	Liver	Heart	Spleen	Lung	Kidney
YANG ORGAN	Gall Bladder	Small Intestine	Stomach	Large Intestine	Bladder
SEASON	Spring	Summer	Late Summer	Autumn	Winter
CLIMATE	Wind	Heat	Damp	Dryness	Cold
COLOUR	Green	Red	Yellow	White	Blue/Black
TASTE	Sour	Bitter	Sweet	Pungent	Salty
SMELL	**Rancid**	**Scorched**	**Fragrant**	**Rotting**	**Putrid**
ORIFICE	Eyes	Tongue	Mouth	Nose	Ears
TISSUE	Tendons	Blood Vessels	Flesh	Skin	Bones
EMOTION	Anger	Over-excitement	Pensiveness	Grief	Fear
VOICE	**Shouting**	**Laughing**	**Singing**	**Weeping**	**Groaning**

Questioning

An important part of a Shiatsu treatment is asking your partner questions. The aim of the questioning is to locate the disharmonies that are causing your partner's symptoms so that you can plan a treatment that will help to correct the imbalance. There is a simple questionnaire (see case-history form on p111) designed to elicit "the signs and symptoms" as well as asking about a person's general health, lifestyle and emotional condition.

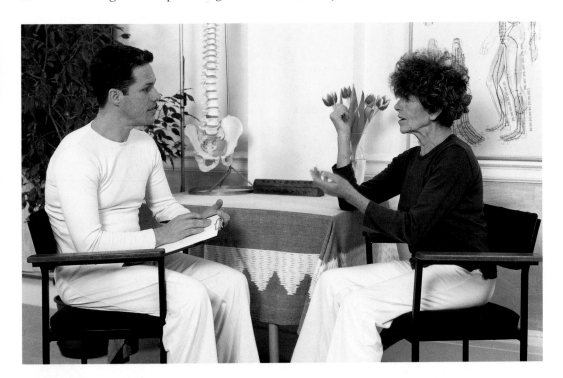

ASSESSING THE SYMPTOMS

When you ask your partner why he or she is seeking a Shiatsu treatment, they will give you an indication of the organ functions that are out of harmony and tell you the health issues they would like addressed. Further questioning may uncover other conditions or symptoms (see box on page 110). All these findings should be carefully noted in a case-history form (see pages 110-11).

TAKING A CASE HISTORY

You need to ask questions that will enable you to assess your partner's condition and decide on what kind of treatment to give. Already you may have made some

Above Set aside five or ten minutes at the beginning of each session to talk to your partner and understand any health issues.

diagnostic assessments relating to their posture, tone of voice or facial characteristics; as you ask questions you can be checking how the answers match up to these initial assessments. It is also important to explain what you are going to do, answer any questions your partner has, reassure them about the treatment and help them to feel relaxed and secure. People often find it hard to talk openly about their problems, so you should always accept what they say without criticizing or judging.

One of the first questions will be about their current conditions. Do they have any symptoms? This question will often be an indicator of the kind of treatment that is expected. For example, if someone is coming to you because they have stiff shoulders, they will expect you to treat their shoulders, and hope to feel better afterwards. As a practitioner you need to address the symptoms that concern your partner, although there may be other areas you want to work on as well.

Asking about emotional states can be difficult. Ask questions such as "Do you suffer from depression or anxiety?" or "Do you find yourself frequently frustrated and irritable?". What you are looking for in their answers is a predominance or an absence of an emotion. It is normal to feel emotional in response to situations, but if someone is always angry or upset, for example, then this shows an imbalance.

SYMPTOM ASSESSMENT CLUES

- Medical history may show a pattern of disharmony in one element. For example, someone who has suffered a bereavement may then frequently suffer from colds and coughs, indicating the Metal element.
- Medication can mask symptoms or produce side effects which can confuse the diagnosis.
- Digestive system problems show a condition in the Earth element. Loose bowels show Spleen deficiency, constipation is linked to Large Intestine. Appetite and eating problems are related to Stomach.
- Diet and taste attraction will give clues as to out-of-balance organs. Someone with a sweet tooth may have other symptoms in Earth, such as loose bowels.
- Excessive drinking of coffee and tea can affect Kidney as caffeine stimulates the production of adrenalin. Alcohol may also affect Liver.
- Menstrual problems and PMS can be signs that Liver is not doing its job of moving chi. Lack of periods can be caused by a deficiency in Spleen.
- Back problems, particularly in the lower back, show Kidney and Bladder imbalances.
- Night-time urination also relates to Kidney and Bladder.
- Breathing difficulties, coughing or frequent colds indicate that the Metal element is out of harmony.
- Headaches, eye problems and stiff joints are all symptoms indicating a Wood imbalance.
- Insomnia or disturbed dreams show Heart imbalance, as do circulation problems such as varicose veins.
- A site of pain may give you an indication of the meridian involved. Note the meridian that passes through or is dominant in this area.
- Energy levels at different times of day will indicate meridian imbalances. For example, if someone is always tired in the morning it indicates a Spleen imbalance.

Finally, you should write down your postural observations, the hara diagnosis and the treatment. Write down any extra changes or symptoms that you noticed. For example, you may have felt that the left shoulder was stiffer than the right, and you could come back to this next time.

In reaching a diagnosis you will be working from your hara diagnosis (see pages 112–13). The case history will help you to confirm your diagnosis or to see deeper underlying patterns. When assessing the case history, look for three or more symptoms or indications in a meridian. You can also use your diagnosis as a basis for any recommendations to your client on self-massage, exercise, diet or lifestyle.

THE CASE-HISTORY FORM

As a professional practitioner you will always need to keep accurate records of your clients' treatments and case notes, so get into the habit as soon as you start treatments of filling in a case-history form such as the one shown opposite. The form should be fully completed at the end of a treatment, although most of it will have been filled in before treatment has started.

When a client returns to you for a further session, you should refer back to the case-history form, to see at-a-glance the symptoms they had when they first came and then, over a period of time, whether or not their condition is improving. The case-history form will also show any significant changes in your diagnosis over successive treatments as well as the overall effectiveness of your treatment.

PREPARING YOUR PARTNER

A Shiatsu treatment will often result in an immediate improvement, but it is also quite normal to feel some adverse reactions. Let your partner know this before you start the treatment, in case they have a sudden reaction during or immediately after the treatment. You can then reiterate this after the treatment (see page 120).

Below Asking questions and listening well to your partner's problems play a central role in Shiatsu diagnosis.

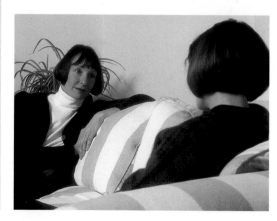

CASE HISTORY

Name:
Address:
Tel. no.:
Occupation:

Reasons for seeking a Shiatsu treatment:

Current symptoms:

Medical history:
(include surgery / major illnesses + when)

Medication currently taking:

Digestive system:
Bowels:
Appetite:

Diet:
Taste attraction:
Coffee / tea / alcohol:

Reproductive system:
Menstruation / PMT:
Back problems:
Chronic / acute where / when:
Urinary system:
Frequency / night:

Respiratory system:
Breathing/coughs:
Smoker:
Headaches / eye problems:
Joints:

Sleep:
Insomnia / dreams:
Circulation:

Energy levels:
Best time of day:
Worst time of day:
Dominant emotion:

Postural observations:

Pain – where / when:

Hara diagnosis (kyo and jitsu):

Treatment notes (treatment carried out / conclusions):

Below The overall treatment process will enable you to focus on individual health problems that need addressing. Often the diagnosis will simply support the symptoms your partner has specified, but sometimes the treatment uncovers other weak areas that need rebalancing – all these must be carefully recorded on the case-history form.

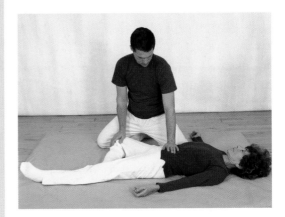

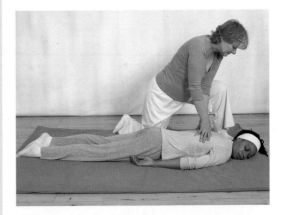

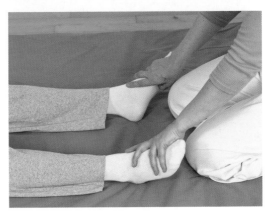

Touching

Touch is the most important diagnostic tool in Shiatsu. When palpating different areas of the body you are using touch to look for areas of kyo (empty) and jitsu (full). Diagnosis requires practice and an empty and receptive mind similar to that reached when meditating – detached, observant and focused. Try not to have any preconceived ideas about the result and remain open, calm and focused.

Hara Diagnosis

Each meridian has a corresponding diagnostic area in the hara. By palpating these areas we can assess for kyo and jitsu. The area with the most empty (kyo) energy state and the one with the most full (jitsu) are the two meridians chosen to work on.

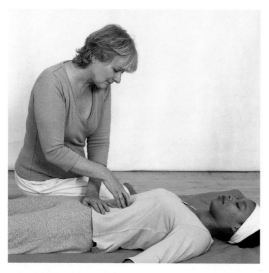

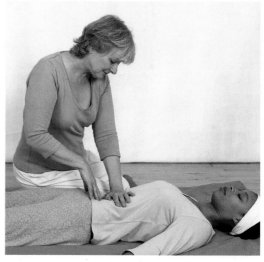

1 Palpate upper hara Leaving the mother hand on the lower hara, palpate the areas in the upper hara with the other (relaxed) hand, using the first three fingers. Follow the steps on the page opposite.

2 Palpate lower hara As you move through the steps, swap the mother hand and place it on the upper hara. Do not press directly into the navel but circle the fingers around it.

Preparing for hara diagnosis
Sit in seiza, close to your partner. Take deep breaths and assess your own state. Observe your partner's energy as you place your mother hand on the lower hara, and the other hand at the side of the belly. Ask yourself "which is the most jitsu area in the hara?" Use a light touch to assess each area, using the same order so that it becomes automatic. Use a cushion to practise.

Checking your diagnosis
When working the channels and points feel for relative kyo and jitsu. Sometimes you can use this to check your diagnosis. Does the meridian you have chosen from the hara diagnosis feel the most kyo meridian? There may be localised areas or points that are kyo or jitsu which relate to a particular condition but don't necessarily reflect the underlying cause and are not the most kyo meridian.

Step-by-step Palpations

The diagram below shows a suggested working sequence for hara diagnosis.
Each of the diagnostic areas in the hara is shown, starting with the Heart and
working gradually round to end with the Small Intestine.

With the mother hand on the lower hara, palpate the areas 1–9 in the upper hara, using the first three fingers and a relaxed hand. Change the mother hand to the upper hara and palpate areas 10–12. Using two hands, fingers pointing down at right angles to the body, work simultaneously on areas 13–14. Where there are two or three areas of the same meridian they should have the same energetic quality. Having moved around the hara quickly, no more than twice, ask the question "which is the most jitsu area?". If you don't know, take a guess and allow your intuition to guide you. Then go round the hara again holding the jitsu area with your mother hand and look for the kyo area, the place that creates a reaction in the jitsu – a softening, a feeling of connection, or some other change.

3 Liver is the pale green area further to the right just below the ribs, where the actual liver is. Continue to move to the right and palpate Liver area. Is it more kyo or more jitsu?

2 Gall Bladder is the purple area on the right below the ribs. Drop your fingers into the Gall Bladder. Is it more kyo or more jitsu than the previous area?

1 Heart is the soft red area at the base of the sternum. With a relaxed hand, using the first three fingers of one hand (the other is the mother hand on the lower abdomen), gently press down, feeling for kyo and jitsu.

4 Lung is the dark grey area further right towards the end of the ribs in the soft area at the waist. Move your relaxed hand to Lung area and again assess for relative kyo and jitsu.

5 Come back to the Heart area (1).

6 Stomach is the yellow area under the left ribs just over the stomach. Continue down the left side palpating the Stomach area.

7 Triple Heater is the pink oval further to the left under the ribs. Palpate Triple Heater area assessing for relative kyo and jitsu. By now you should have a most kyo and a most jitsu area.

8 Lung is the dark grey circle on the left, matching the right Lung area in step 4. Try to remember how it felt on the right side and compare. Return to these two areas again at the end, using two hands to compare.

9 Heart Protector is the deep red oval on the mid-line between the base of the sternum and the navel, just below the top Heart area. Gently palpate with three fingers, looking for relative kyo and jitsu.

10 Spleen is the mid-brown area around the navel. Move the mother hand to above the navel. Use the three fingers and your thumb around the navel. Avoid pressing into the navel directly.

11 Kidney is the blue horseshoe-shaped area below and around the sides of the navel. Palpate below the navel and then use two hands to feel the horseshoe sides.

12 Bladder is the pale blue outer horseshoe. Palpate just above the pubic bone and with two hands round the sides.

Key to the meridians

- Small Intestine
- Triple Heater
- Large Intestine
- Stomach
- Lung
- Heart
- Heart Protector
- Liver
- Spleen
- Kidney
- Gall Bladder
- Bladder

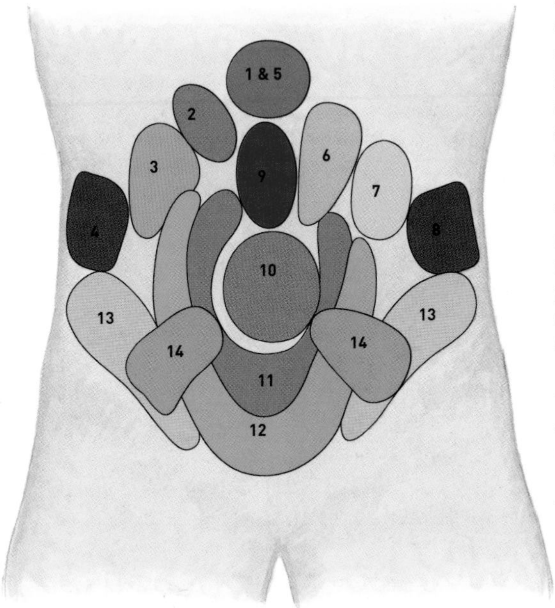

14 Small Intestine areas are the egg shapes superimposed over the Large Intestine, Bladder and Kidney. Palpate with two hands, comparing energetic quality and seeing if they have the same fullness or emptiness.

13 Large Intestine areas are pale grey flat ovals above each hip bone. Work with two hands.

Planning a Treatment

Having done all the background work setting up a Shiatsu treatment room and organizing loose cotton clothing (see page 46), you'll then need to come up with a treatment structure that suits you. The session should always include diagnosis using all the different methods, followed by the hands-on treatment (taking into account the contraindications listed on page 47) and some time afterwards for recovery.

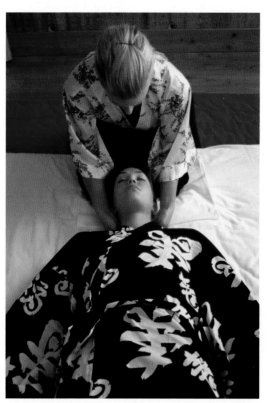

Above Both partners should wear comfortable, loose cotton clothing that covers as much as possible (Shiatsu treatments should not be carried out on exposed skin) and treatment should be on a firm, but soft, base such as a futon.

Right Always start every Shiatsu session with a hara diagnosis. Make a note of any full or empty areas, and return to the hara to feel for any changes as you progress. Having completed the diagnosis, Shiatsu practitioners generally work first on the kyo meridian: this helps to relax the jitsu and address the cause of the energy imbalance.

TREATMENT STRUCTURE

Start by following the basic framework outline in your treatments (see pages 44–67), starting with a hara diagnosis and slotting in the relevant meridians when you come to the arms or legs. As you become more experienced you can change the order of your treatment. You could start with a hara diagnosis, then work on the front of the body on the arms or legs, according to which meridians you have chosen. In some cases it is better to start working on the back after the hara diagnosis, especially if your receiver has not had Shiatsu before, as it is more relaxing.

Usually the actual hands-on treatment lasts about 35 to 40 minutes. This gives time at the beginning to take a case history and form a diagnosis and 5 minutes at the end for your partner to recover and for you to give them any recommendations you may have (see page 120). So altogether the treatment should take an hour from start to finish. When you are just beginning, it will almost certainly take longer, but with practice you should be able to hone down the treatment time to an hour.

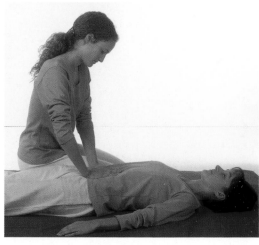

A Simple Treatment Sequence

Your treatment structure should always include work on the Bladder meridian, because of its relation to the spine and the nervous system. There are points on Bladder meridian either side of the spine that have a direct effect on each of the organ functions, known as yu points.

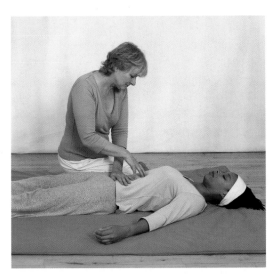

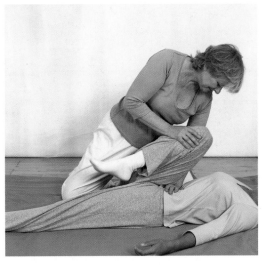

1 Hara diagnosis Sit in seiza position next to your partner's abdomen, placing your hand on the hara and tuning into your partner's energy. Do a hara diagnosis, moving quickly round the hara. Use the diagnosis as a focus for your treatment.

2 Leg rotation In this treatment we are using Spleen kyo, Lung jitsu as a diagnosis. Work the kyo meridian first – in this case Spleen. Start with leg rotation, keeping your hand on the hara and feeling for any stiffness in the hips.

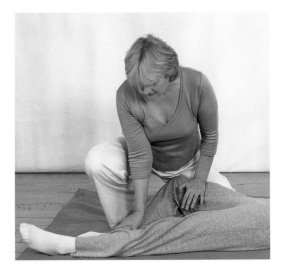

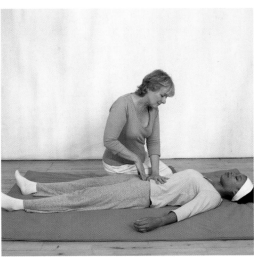

3 Palm the meridian Drop the leg down, lifting your own leg to kneel forward. Rest your partner's knee on your thigh for extra support if needed. Work the meridian with your palm and then your thumb, as shown on page 48.

4 Reassess hara energy Return to a seiza position next to the hara as you draw back the leg and complete the Spleen meridian. Feel the difference in the energy in the hara: has it altered since you started the Shiatsu sequence?

▷

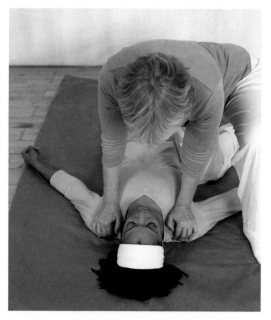

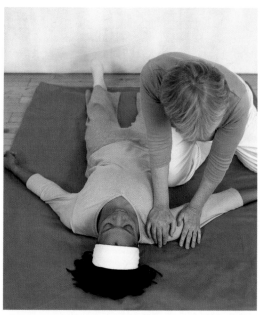

5 Open up the chest Move up to the shoulders by stepping up with one leg so that your foot is in line with your partner's shoulder. Place your hands on each shoulder and lean in with your body weight to open up the chest.

6 Thumb down Put the arm at 45 degrees – the position to treat the Lung meridian. With your mother hand firmly on the shoulder, palm and then thumb down the Lung meridian from the shoulder to the wrist.

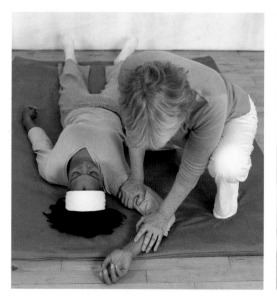

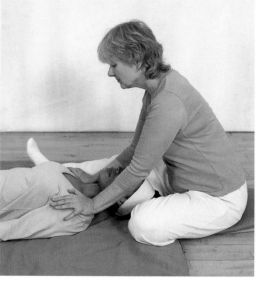

7 Open up the shoulder Holding the wrist, step up and bring the arm over the head. With your hand on the shoulder stretch the arm and open up the shoulder. Turn so that you are facing the feet in a position ready to work the head and neck.

8 Pressure on shoulders Replace your partner's arms by their sides and move above the head. Adopt a relaxed seiza position with one leg straight for balance. Place your hands on the shoulders, pointing down the body, and apply pressure.

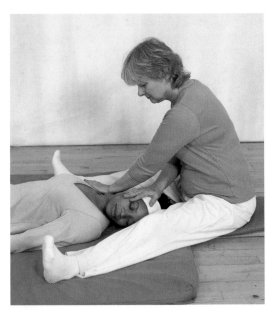

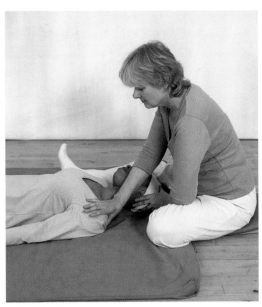

9 Rotate head Place one hand on the side of the head, the other on the shoulder and rotate the head, turning the chin towards the opposite shoulder. Open up the side of the neck by stretching the two hands away from each other.

10 Head to the side Side bend the head by placing one hand on the side of the head and the other on the shoulder. Push the head sideways, away from the shoulder you are holding, to open up the neck. Repeat on the other side.

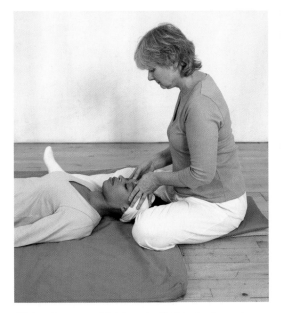

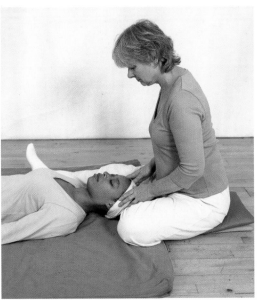

11 Thumb pressure Find the point BL 2, in the depression under the inner end of the eyebrow ridge. This point can be painful, so apply gentle but focused pressure with your thumbs making sure they are perpendicular to your partner's face.

12 Thumbing up Continue in a straight line from BL 2, thumbing up Bladder meridian in the forehead and over and behind the head as far as you can reach. These last two techniques are good to release tension in the eyes and head. ▷

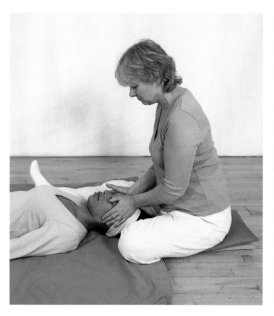

13 Palming head Palm around the top of the head with the heel of your hand. This covers the Gall Bladder meridian, which goes over the head several times. It is an important pathway for chi energy to circulate and activate the brain.

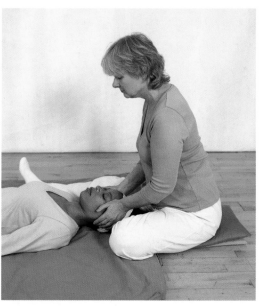

14 Rest head Bring your fingertips under the base of the skull and allow the head to rest in the palms of your hands. Come around to the other side and repeat the arm and leg sequence on the other side.

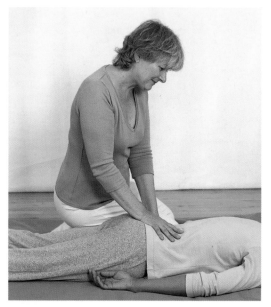

15 Assess energy flow Turn your partner over into prone position. Centre yourself by placing your hands on the sacrum. Tune in to the chi energy flow, feeling for any signs of fullness (jitsu) or emptiness (kyo).

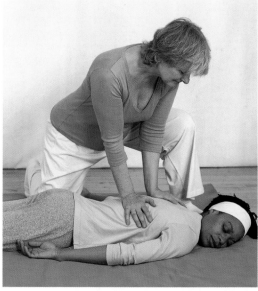

16 Palm down Step up with one leg forward and palm down Bladder meridian in the back, starting one hand's width below the neck. Notice any over- or under-energized areas as you work down. Finish when you reach the sacrum.

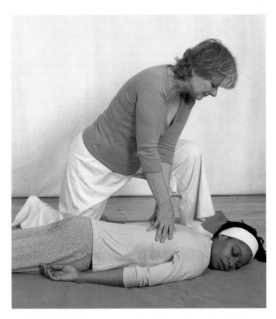

17 Thumb down Come back to the top and thumb down the Bladder meridian two finger-widths either side of the mid-line. Use perpendicular pressure leaning in with your weight. Notice kyo or jitsu points.

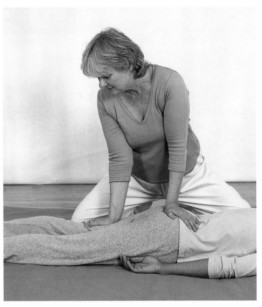

18 Palm down When you have completed Bladder in the back, turn to face the body and with mother hand on the sacrum and a wide seiza position, palm down the back of the leg. Shift your position down the leg as you work down.

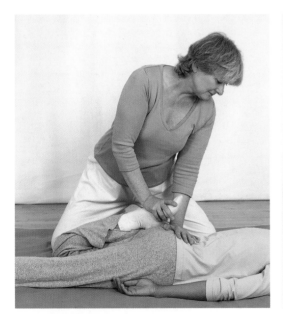

19 Stretch foot When you reach the ankle, pick up the leg under the ankle and stretch the foot to the buttock. Keep your hand on the sacrum and be careful not to over-stretch. Replace the leg and work down the other leg.

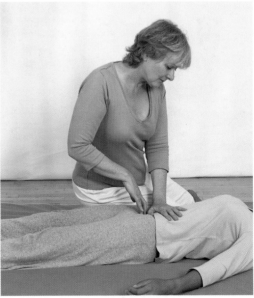

20 Hara assessment Turn your partner back over into supine position. Sit in seiza by the hara and check to see if there has been a change. Let your hand rest on the hara to finish, slowly breaking contact.

Finishing a Session

Having finished the physical Shiatsu treatment, first let your partner relax. Then remind them about how the treatment may affect them, alerting them to any ways that they may feel different, and offer yourself as a source of support if they are concerned by their physical or emotional reaction. Finally, complete the case history of their lifestyle patterns and the treatment that you carried out.

RELAXATION

After coming back to the hara to check whether it has changed, allow your partner to lie still for a few minutes to enjoy the feeling of deep relaxation and balance and allow the body to process any changes that have occurred. You may want to leave the room to allow your partner to be alone, and give yourself recovery time too.

TREATMENT REACTIONS

At the end of a treatment warn your partner that they should expect some changes over the following hours or days. Mostly they will feel better immediately, but it is quite common to feel tired, and you should advise them to have a rest if they do. Some people may have a headache or feel emotional, and this is also normal. Sometimes when the body's energy is changing it may be felt as discomfort. Encourage your partner to contact you for advice if conditions or problems develop.

Below Makka-ho exercises help to activate the meridians and are easy to do yourself at home – this one is a simple exercise to help the Spleen and Stomach meridians.

The effects of treatment

The immediate effect of Shiatsu treatment is individual, and partly depends on the length and depth of the treatment. A sense of well-being is common. The time taken for relief of symptoms depends on the nature of the condition. Because of the deep relaxation that usually occurs and the stimulus to the major body systems, your partner may experience "healing reactions": flu-like symptoms, aches, changes in bowel movements and urination, headaches or low energy may appear for around 24 hours. These are signs of elimination and show that healing is beginning.

If your partner suffers any serious adverse effects after treatment, he or she should seek medical help. If it is a more mild reaction, use the following guidelines:
• Take it easy and do not exert the body unnecessarily
• Avoid caffeine, alcohol and other drugs
• Take a lot of rest and go to bed earlier than usual
• Relax in a warm bath to sweat out some of the toxins
• Eat plenty of fresh fruit and vegetables, preferably raw
• Drink plenty of fresh water and hot water
• Avoid sugary and fatty foods

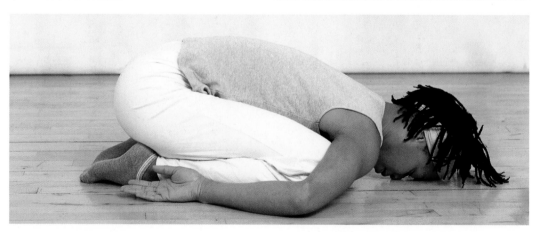

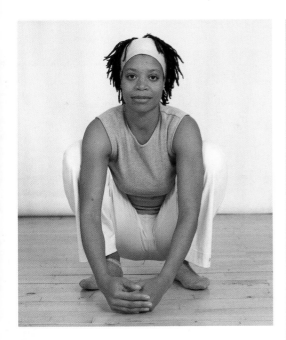

Above This makka-ho squatting exercise increases flexibility in the hips, knees and ankles. Be aware of your hara and let your weight drop into the feet from the belly.

RECOMMENDATIONS

Suggesting some simple recommendations will help your partner to continue the healing process. These may include activities, such as dancing, T'ai Chi or sports. You can teach them one or two of the makka-ho exercises described on pages 40–3 to help activate specific meridians. These are simple to do and can be applied to a particular condition. For example, if your partner has a problem with digestion or appetite you could recommend the Stomach/Spleen makka-ho exercise described on page 41. Or if your partner's emotions need bringing into balance, use the stretch on page 42 that works on the Heart and Small Intestine. If you want to give dietary advice, then keep it very simple or recommend a nutritionist. Look at the five elements correspondences table on pages 122–3 to see the taste attraction. If you have treated Spleen or Stomach, you could suggest substituting fruit or sweet vegetables for sugar. Restrict your advice to one or two recommendations that your partner can easily achieve; sooner choose something positive that can be added to a lifestyle, rather than something to give up. Don't be afraid to recommend other kinds of practitioners with more expertise in a particular area. Get to know some practitioners, such as counsellors, reflexologists, acupuncturists, homeopaths and herbalists, whom you feel confident to recommend.

Recommendations by element

An important part of every Shiatsu treatment is to give recommendations for suitable follow-up exercises to work on and lifestyle changes to be introduced. It can give your partner a real sense of empowerment to know that they can make changes to improve a condition. Make a point of giving simple recommendations that your partner can feasibly achieve.

EARTH – SPLEEN AND STOMACH MERIDIANS
- Dietary modification and measures for losing weight:
  Chewing each mouthful slowly (10 – 30 times)
  Eating a good breakfast
  Making meal times relaxed and stress free
- Grounding exercises such as T'ai Chi and Chi Kung
- Getting nourishment or pampering from sources other than food, such as music, receiving Shiatsu or other types of massage

FIRE – HEART AND SMALL INTESTINE, HEART PROTECTOR AND TRIPLE HEATER
- Meditation or relaxation tapes to calm the shen
- Skin brushing to improve the circulation
- Singing to encourage expression
- Counselling for emotional problems

METAL – LUNG AND LARGE INTESTINE
- Breathing exercises to encourage the taking in of chi
- Any vigorous exercise or a sport to encourage the intake of oxygen and to be more social
- Yoga to help with breathing
- Getting out of the house – going to a film, theatre or dancing – for a change of environment

WATER – KIDNEY AND BLADDER
Rest and moderation are important as Water people tend to overdo everything and become exhausted.
- Meditation is often difficult for a Water person to do, but they could try more active types of meditation, such as visualization or autogenic training
- Coffee over-stimulates the kidneys and cutting down or drinking decaffeinated coffee can help
- Alcohol and recreational drugs are particularly damaging

WOOD – LIVER AND GALL BLADDER
Wood people will often be workaholics and tend to be overly controlling.
- Encourage a good balance between work and play
- Creative pursuits such as pottery, writing, drawing etc.
- Non-competitive sport or outdoor activities, such as swimming, walking or gardening
- Dancing is excellent for encouraging flexibility, grace and self-expression

Five Elements Correspondences Table

	WOOD	FIRE
Yin organ	Liver	Heart Heart Protector
Yang organ	Gall Bladder	Small Intestine Triple Heater
Colour	Green	Red / Purple
Voice	Shouting	Laughing
Negative emotion	Anger Frustration	Excitement Hysteria
Positive emotion	Patience Humour	Calmness
Taste	Sour	Bitter
Smell	Rancid	Scorched
Sense	Sight	Speech
Orifice/body part	Eyes	Tongue
Season	Spring	Summer
Time of day	11 p.m. – 3 a.m.	11 p.m. – 3 a.m. 7 p.m. – 11 p.m.
Damaging climate	Wind	Heat
Body tissue	Tendons Ligaments	Blood vessels
Function	Organization Decisions	Consciousness Communication
Fluid secretion	Tears	Sweat
System	Joints	Circulation
Direction	East	South
Spirit	Life direction	Consciousness
Stage of development	Birth	Growth
Nurturing foods	Wheat Leafy green vegetables	Corn (sweetcorn) Beans

EARTH	METAL	WATER
Spleen	Lung	Kidney
Stomach	Large Intestine	Bladder
Yellow / Orange	White	Blue / Black
Singing Whining	Weeping	Groaning
Worry Victim	Grief Isolated	Fear Phobias
Compassion Grounded	Positive Open	Courage
Sweet	Pungent	Salty
Fragrant	Rotting	Putrid
Taste	Smell	Hearing
Mouth	Nose	Ears
Late summer	Autumn	Winter
7 a.m. – 11 a.m.	3 a.m. – 7 a.m.	3 p.m. – 7 p.m.
Damp	Dryness	Cold
Flesh	Skin Membranes	Bones Hair
Transformation Transportation	Exchange Elimination	Purification Regulation
Saliva	Mucus	Urine
Digestive	Respiratory Eliminatory	Nervous Reproductive
Centre	West	North
Intellect	Soul	Will
Transformation	Harvest	Hibernation
Rice Root vegetables	Lotus root Ginger	Millet Aduki beans

Useful Addresses

UK

The Shiatsu Society (UK)
Eastlands Court
St Peters Rd
Rugby CV21 3QP
Tel: +44 8451 304560
www.shiatsu.org

British School of Shiatsu-Do
Unit 3
Islington Studios
Thane Villas
London N7 7NV
Tel: +44 20 770 03355
www.shiatsu-do.co.uk

USA

AOBTA National Headquarters
1010 Haddonfield-Berlin Road
Suite 408
Voorhees, NJ 08043-3514
Tel: 856 782 1616
www.aobta.org

International School of Shiatsu
10 South Clinton Street
Doylestown, PA 18901
Tel: 215 340 9918
Fax: 215 340 9181
Email:info@shiatsubo.com
www.shiatsubo.com

Ohashi Institute
147 West 25th St
8th Floor
New York, NY 10001
Tel: 800 810 4190
Email: info@ohashiatsu.org
www.ohashi.com

Canada

The Canadian Shiatsu Society of
British Columbia (CSSBC)
www.Shiatsupractor.org

Shiatsu School of Canada Inc.
547 College Street, Toronto
Ontario, M6G 1A9
Tel: 416 323-1818

or toll-free: 1 800 263 1703
Fax: 416 323 1681
Email: info@shiatsucanada.com
www.shiatsucanada.com

Shiatsu Academy of Tokyo
320 Danforth Avenue, Suite 206
Toronto, Ontario M4K 1N8
Tel: 416 466 8780
Email: sait131@aol.com
www.kensensaito.com

Sourcepoint Shiatsu Therapy Centre
3261 Heather Street (at 16th Ave.)
Vancouver, British Columbia V5Z 3K4
Tel: 604 876 0042
Fax: 604 876 3398
Email: info@sourcepoint.bc.ca
www.sourcepoint.bc.ca

Australia

Shiatsu Academy
54 Brighton Road
Balaclava
Melbourne, Victoria 3183
Tel: 03 9525 7968
Fax: 03 9525 7968

Shiatsu Therapy Association
of Australia
c/o The Secretary
PO Box 91
Brunswick West, Victoria 305
Tel: 03 9380 9183 or 1300 138 250
www.staa.org.au

New Zealand

Tao Shiatsu Oceania
9 Hemington St, Waterview, Auckland
Tel: 09 828 3385
Mob: 025 989 726
Email: oceania@taoshiatsu.com
www.taoshiatsu.com

Japan

Japan Shiatsu College
2-15-6 Koishikawa, Bunkyo-ku Tokyo
Tel: 03 3813 7481
www.shiatsu.ac.jp

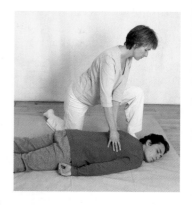

Europe

The European Shiatsu
Federation
www.shiatsu-esf.org

Austria

Österreichischer Dachverband für
Shiatsu
Postfach 109, A-1217 Wien
Tel/fax: +43 1 258 08 49
Email: info@shiatsu-verband.at
www.shiatsu-verband.at

Belgium

Belgische Shiatsu Federatie vzw
Gounden Leeuwplein 1
B-9000 Gent
Tel: +32 92 252 904
Email: info@shiatsu.be
www.shiatsu.be

Czech Republic

CAS Czech Shiatsu Association
Na Zderaze 5
120 00 Praha 2
Tel: +42 0603 156 708
Email: darja@shiatsu.cz

Greece

Hellenic Shiatsu Society
Zissimopoulou 16
115-24 Athens
Tel: +30 (0) 10 6980 168
Email: mcharl@tee.gr

Holland

Iokai Shiatsu Akademie
  Nederland
1E Jacob Van Campenstr. 40
BG Amsterdam
1072 Netherlands
Email: info@iokai-shiatsu.nl
www.iokai-shiatsu.nl

Ireland

Shiatsu Society of Ireland
P.O. Box 7683,
Malahide, Co. Dublin
Tel: +353 1 845 3647
www.shiatsusocietyireland.com

Israel

Israeli Tao Shiatsu Center
Tzvika Calisar
Spinoza 5, Tel-Aviv
Tel: 03 524 9277
Email: Europe@taoshiatsu.com
www.taoshiatsu.co.il

Spain

Asociación de Profesionales de
  Shiatsu en España
C/ Atocha, 121-1°-izda
E-28012 Madrid
Tel/fax: +34 91 429 49 89
Email: Shiastu@terra.es
www.shiatsu-es.com

Sweden

Riksorganisationen för Shiatsu
Rusthållarvägen 6
S-18769 Täby
Tel: +46 8 766 40 05
Email: info@shiatsuriks.org
www.shiatsuriks.org

Switzerland

International School of Shiatsu
Hauptstrasse
Kiental / BE
CH 3723
Tel: +41 33 676 26 76
www.kientalerhof.ch

Acknowledgements

Author's Acknowledgements

I would like to thank my editor Jennifer Mussett for encouraging me and, in difficult circumstances, helping me in the completion of this book. My heartfelt thanks go to all my teachers who have inspired me in this journey into the wondrous working of the human body and its energy patterns, especially to my first teachers Ray Ridolfi, Saul Goodman, Pauline Sasaki and Ohashi Sensei.

I would like to acknowledge my fellow teachers and students at the British School of Shiatsu-Do for the fund of knowledge that they have shared, which forms the basis of this book. Special thanks to Maura Bright for information on facial diagnosis and to Doe Warnes, Emerson Bastos, Kishaw Wheatle, Maya Babic, Cynthia Kee and Cesar Pinto for their patience and enthusiasm as the models. To Katy Bevan for organizing us all and first suggesting that I do this book.

I am deeply grateful to all my teachers, colleagues, students and clients who have shared this Shiatsu path with me – for all the healing, friendship, inspiration and support.

My special thanks to my two children Layla and Talal who have loved and supported me unconditionally and without whose father, Edward Totah, I would never have started on this road.

Publisher's Acknowledgements

The publishers would like to thank the following for permission to reproduce their images: p11 Charles Pertwee/Alamy Images, p71m Image source/Alamy, p114 image100/Alamy; p12, p13 Mary Evans Picture Library; p49tr Robert Harding Picture Library. All other photographs © Anness Publishing

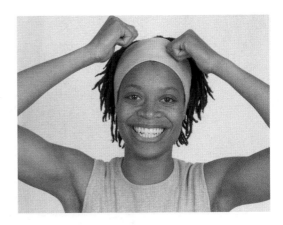

Index

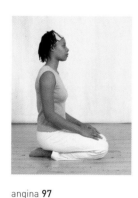
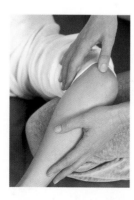
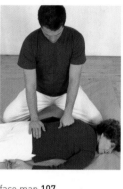
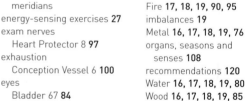

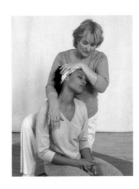

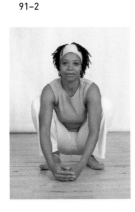

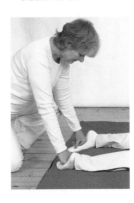

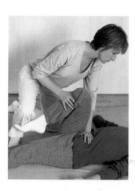

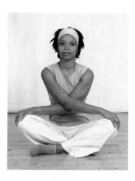

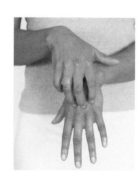

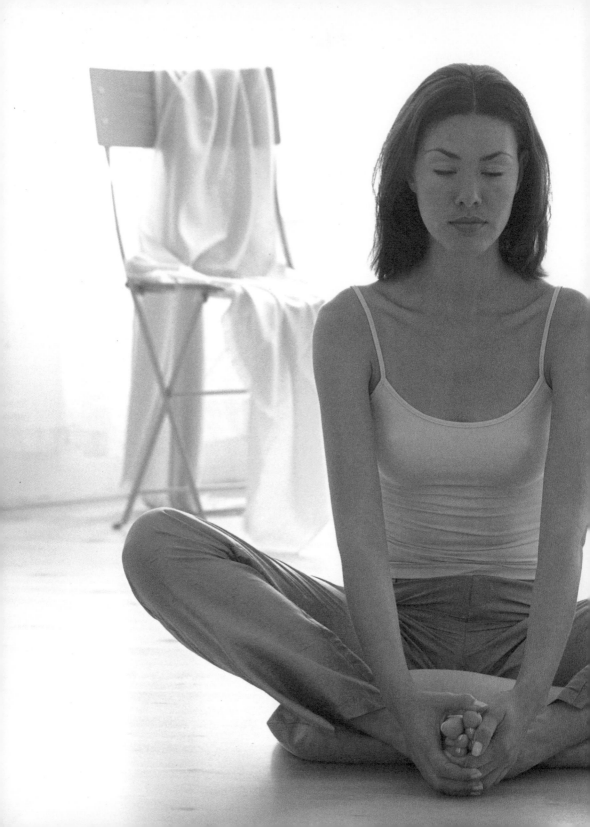